Carbohydrates in human nutrition

FAO FOOD AND
NUTRITION
PAPER

66

Report of a Joint FAO/WHO Expert Consultation
Rome, 14-18 April 1997

**WORLD
HEALTH
ORGANIZATION**

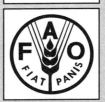

**Food
and
Agriculture
Organization
of
the
United
Nations**

Rome, 1998

Reprinted 1998

M-86
ISBN 92-5-104114-8

CONTENTS

TABLES

FIGURES

ANNEXES

TABLES

TABLES

FIGURES

Acknowledgements

FAO and WHO express their gratitude for the contribution of the experts who participated in this consultation and contributed to the development of the report. The organizations are also thankful for those participating as well as non-participating experts who have prepared draft background papers in the preparatory process for the consultation. Extracts of those papers have been used in creating the background information included in Annex 2 of the report. Special appreciation is offered to Dr. David Lineback and Dr. Ruth Oniang'o, who served as the Chairman and Vice-Chair, respectively, and to Drs. Thomas Wolever and Mark Wahlqvist who jointly undertook the demanding task of acting as Rapporteurs for the Consultation.

Participants

Nils-Georg ASP
Chemical Centre
University of Lund
P.O. Box 124
22100 Lund
Sweden

John CUMMINGS
MRC Dunn Clinical Nutrition Centre
Hills Road
Cambridge CB2 2DH
United Kingdom

Erik Osvaldo DIAZ BUSTOS
Department of Nutrition
Faculty of Medicine
University of Chile
Casilla 138-11
Santiago 11
Chile

Mark DREHER
Nutrition and Scientific Regulatory Affairs
Nabisco, Inc.
Technology Center
200 DeForest Avenue
East Hanover, NJ 07936-1944
USA

Mukund GURJAR
Indian Institute of Chemical Technology
Council of Scientific and Industrial
Research, Government of India
Hyderabad 500 007
India

Seyed Masoud KIMIAGAR
National Nutrition Institute
Dean, Nutrition and Food Science College
P.O. Box 19395/4741
Tehran
Islamic Republic of Iran

Shuhei KOBAYASHI
The National Institute of Health and
Nutrition
1-23-1, Toyama, Shinjuku-ku
Tokyo 162
Japan

David LINEBACK (*Chairman*)
College of Agriculture
University of Idaho.
Moscow, Idaho, 83844-2331
USA

James I. MANN
Professor of Human Nutrition
University of Otago
P.O.Box 56
Dunedin
New Zealand

Ruth ONIANG'O (*Vice-Chair*)
Director
Board of Postgraduate Studies
Jomo Kenyatta University of Agriculture
and Technology
P.O. Box 62000
Nairobi
Kenya

James HILL
Center of Human Nutrition
University of Colorado Health Science
Center
4200 East Ninth Avenue
Campus Box C225
Denver, Colorado 80262
USA

Kraisid TONTISIRIN
Institute of Nutrition
Mahidol University
Salaya, Phutthamonthon 4
Nakhon Pathom 73170
Thailand

Hester Hendrina VORSTER
Potchefstroom University for Christian
Higher Education
Dept. of Nutrition and Family Ecology
Private Bag X6001
Potchefstroom 2520
Republic of South Africa

Alison STEPHEN
Division of Nutrition and Dietetics
College of Pharmacy and Nutrition
University of Saskatchewan
110 Science Place
Saskatoon, Saskatchewan, S7N 5C9
Canada

Mark WAHLQVIST
Monash Medical Centre
Monash University
246 Clayton Road
Clayton, Melbourne
Victoria 3168
Australia

Thomas WOLEVER
Department of Nutritional Sciences
University of Toronto
150 College Street
Toronto, Ontario, M5S 3E2
Canada

Secretariat

FOOD AND AGRICULTURE
ORGANIZATION OF THE
UNITED NATIONS

Guy NANTEL
Senior Officer
Nutrition Planning, Assessment and
Evaluation Service
Food and Nutrition Division
FAO, Rome

John R. WEATHERWAX
Consultant to FAO, Rome.

WORLD HEALTH
ORGANIZATION

Ratko BUZINA
Consultant, Nutrition
WHO, Geneva

Graeme CLUGSTON
Director, Nutrition Programme
WHO, Geneva.

Nicolai KHALTAEV
Responsible Officer
Chronic Noncommunicable Diseases.
WHO, Geneva

Contributors

Nils-Georg ASP
Department of Applied Nutrition and
Food Chemistry
Chemical Centre, University of Lund
Lund
Sweden.

Inger BJÖRK
Department of Applied Nutrition and
Food Chemistry, Chemical Centre,
University of Lund, Lund
Sweden.

Christine CHERBUT
Human Nutrition Research Centre,
Institut National de la Recherche
Agronomique
Nantes
France

Mark DREHER
Scientific Nutrition Affairs
Nabisco Inc.
New Jersey
USA.

James HILL
Center for Human Nutrition,
University of Colorado Health Science
Center
Denver, Colorado, USA.

M. HILL
European Cancer Prevention
Organization, Lady Sobell
Gastrointestinal Unit
Wexham Park Hospital
Slough, Berkshire
United Kingdom

Megha LAL
Division of Nutrition and Dietetics,
College of Pharmacy and Nutrition,
University of Saskatchewan,
Saskatoon, Saskatchewan
Canada.

Ronald LAUER
Division of Pediatric Cardiology
University of Iowa
Iowa City, Iowa
USA

Michael LENTZE
Zentrum für Kinderheilkunde
Bonn
Germany

David LINEBACK
College of Agriculture
University of Idaho
Idaho
USA.

James MANN
University of Otago
Dunedin
New Zealand.

Margareta NYMAN
Department of Applied Nutrition and
Food Chemistry
Chemical Centre, University of Lund,
Lund
Sweden

Klaus KÖNIG
Faculty of Medical Sciences
University of Nijmegen
Nijmegen
The Netherlands.

Leon PROSKY
Prosky Associates
Nutrition Consultants
Rockville, MD
USA.

Barbara ROLLS
Nutrition Department
Pennsylvania State University,
University Park, PA
USA.

Clyde WILLIAMS
Sports Science
Loughborough University
Leicestershire
UK

Alison STEPHEN
Division of Nutrition and Dietetics,
College of Pharmacy and Nutrition,
University of Saskatchewan,
Saskatoon, Saskatchewan
Canada

Thomas WOLEVER
Department of Nutritional Sciences
and Division of Endocrinology and
Metabolism, St. Michael's Hospital,
Univerity of Toronto
Toronto, Ontario
Canada.

Hester VORSTER
Lipid Clinic and Nutrition Research,
Department of Nutrition and Family
Ecology, Potchefstroom University,
Potchefstroom
South Africa.

Mark WOLRAICH
Vanderbilt University Medical Center,
Nashville, TN
USA

Mark WAHLQVIST
Monash University
Monash Medical Centre
Medbourne
Australia.

Reviewers

Harvey ANDERSON
Nutritional Sciences Department
University of Toronto
150 College Street
Toronto, Ontario M5S 3E2
Canada

David BENTON
Department of Psychology
University of Wales Swansea
Singleton Park,
Swansea SA2 8PP
United Kingdom

Mark BIEBER
Nutrition Research Associate
Best Foods
CPC International Inc.
150 Pierce St, Call Box 6710
Sommerset NJ 08873-6710
USA

George BLACKBURN
Division of Surgical Nutrition
Deaconess Hospital
Harvard Medical School
One Deaconess Rd
Boston, MA 02215
USA

Eric JEQUIER
Institut de Physiologie
Universit© de Lausanne
Rue de Bugnon 7
CH - 1005 Lausanne
Switzerland

Maurice LESSOFF
8 John Spencer Square
London NW1 2LZ
United Kingdom

Dean METCALFE
Laboratory of Allergic Diseases
National Institute of Allergy and
Infectious Diseases
National Institutes of Health (Bldg. 10)
10 Center Dr MSC 1881
Bethesda MD 20892-1881
USA

Denis O'MULLANE
Department of Preventive and
Paediatric Dentistry
University Dental School and Hospital
Wilton, Cork
Ireland

Marcel ROBERFROID
Université Catholique de Louvain (UCL)
Tour Van Helmont
Avenue E. Mounier, 73
B-1200 Brussels
Belgium

Wim SARIS
Faculty of Health Sciences
Department of Human Biology
University of Maastricht
P.O.Box 616
6200 MDMaastricht
The Netherlands

PREFACE

Carbohydrates are the single most important source of food energy in the world. They comprise some 40 to 80 percent of total food energy intake, depending on locale, cultural considerations or economic status. Those persons with high carbohydrate diets are often in the lower economic strata as foods high in carbohydrate, such as cereal grains, are most often the least expensive. Rice is an excellent example and is the primary staple in the diet of much of the world's population.

Food carbohydrates are not only an energy source, however, they have other roles as well. Typically, sugars are used as sweeteners to make food more palatable and to assist in food preservation. Diets high in carbohydrate may reduce individual propensity to obesity, and there is some evidence that such diets may also provide some protection against various non-communicable human diseases and conditions.

The concept of dietary fibre has changed. Fibre was originally described as plant cell wall material which simply passed through the gut unchanged and provided bulk to feces. Today it is known as an important moderator of digestion in the small bowel and as a major substrate for fermentation in the colon, where the non-starch polysaccharides of the plant cell wall are metabolized to short chain fatty acids. Absorption of the latter provides some energy. In addition, it has been shown that other carbohydrates are present in the diet which enter the colon and are fermented, including resistant starch and non-digestible oligosaccharides.

A previous Joint Expert Consultation on Carbohydrates in Human Nutrition, held in 1979, was wide ranging in scope. The report of that consultation (1) is essentially a reference document outlining the knowledge at that time of the various roles that carbohydrates have in the human diet. Included were the effects of processing on carbohydrates as well as carbohydrate digestion, absorption and metabolism. Of special concern to the consultation were the diets of infants and children. That consultation reached several conclusions regarding each of the areas discussed, and made a number of recommendations for future work.

The Joint FAO/WHO Expert Consultation on Carbohydrates in Human Nutrition was held in Rome from 14 to 18 April 1997. The Consultation was opened by Dr. H. de Haen, Assistant Director-General, Economic and Social Department, FAO, who welcomed the participants on behalf of the Directors-General of FAO and WHO.

In welcoming the participants, Dr. de Haen recalled the previous joint consultation on this subject, which was held in Geneva in 1979. That and the present Consultation are part of a long series of such expert consultations which have as a primary objective the review of the state of knowledge on the role of various nutrients in the human diet and the formulation of practical recommendations where interpretation is needed or controversy exists. The most recent in this series was the Joint FAO/WHO Expert Consultation on Fats and Oils in Human Nutrition held in Rome in 1993.

Consultations such as this are part of a continuing commitment by both FAO and WHO to promote a reliable, nutritious and safe food supply and to provide scientifically sound nutritional advice to member nations. This commitment was recently reaffirmed at the World Food Summit held in November 1996 in Rome.

Dr. de Haen pointed out that the understanding of the role that carbohydrates play in human nutrition and health has made great strides in the 18 years since the previous carbohydrate consultation. Progress in carbohydrate chemistry has permitted the development of a variety of new food products, many of which are based on improved nutritional considerations. Perhaps the greatest impact of recent knowledge is our growing understanding of the diverse physiological roles that carbohydrates have, depending to a great extent on the site, rate and extent of their digestion and fermentation in the gut. This is leading to new dietary approaches, not only for better nutrition, but for improved health as well. Another understanding which has come about in recent years is the influence of carbohydrates on physical performance through glycogen loading. This technique is now well-established as an important factor for the improvement of endurance performance and capacity.

With these new advances in carbohydrate understanding come new issues which have important implications for agricultural production, the food industry and public health policy. Dr. de Haen pointed out that this Consultation will be addressing a number of these issues, and underlined the importance of the Consultation in providing international guidance in this broad area.

Dr. de Haen reminded the participants that they had been invited to the Consultation as independent experts and that their participation in the Consultation was to be in their individual capacity and not as a representative of any organization, affiliation or government.

Dr. Graeme Clugston, Director, WHO Nutrition Programmes, added his welcome to the participants, on behalf of the Director-General of WHO. Dr. Clugston pointed out that the formulation and implementation of science-based dietary guidelines have become a central issue for the nutritional sciences, as well as a major challenge for governments world wide, especially since the International Conference on Nutrition held in Rome, December 1992.

Research during the last two decades has firmly established that diet is one of the major risk factors in the development of a spectrum of non-communicable diseases. Dr. Clugston outlined some of the critical issues in this area, including the roles of mono- and di-saccharides and starch as distinct from non-starch polysaccharides, their relation with dietary fats, and their contribution to dietary energy intakes. Obesity, non-insulin dependent diabetes, coronary heart disease, some cancers (notably colocrectal) and other gastrointestinal tract conditions are among the diseases which can be beneficially influenced by dietary carbohydrates. However, frequent consumption of sugar and other fermentable carbohydrates throughout the day increases the cariogenic risk potential of the diet, especially in the absence of reasonable oral hygienic paractices. On the other hand, sugar intake plays a less important role in caries causation if fluoridation and hygienic measures have been taken.

Dr. Clugston expressed confidence that this Expert Consultation would lead to scientifically sound, up-to-date, pragmatic recommendations on carbohydrates in human nutrition. FAO and WHO would then ensure that these recommendations would be passed on to all member states world wide, providing them with the best possible guidance for developing their own appropriate dietary guidelines for health promotion, good nutrition and disease prevention.

The Consultation elected Dr. David Lineback as Chairman and Dr. Ruth Oniang'o as Vice-Chair. Dr. Mark Wahlquist and Dr. Thomas Wolever were appointed jointly as Rapporteurs. Dr. Lineback in his response indicated the importance of this Consultation and outlined the scope of the issues that would be discussed and on which the two agencies, FAO and WHO, were seeking expert guidance from the Consultation.

CHAPTER 1

THE ROLE OF CARBOHYDRATES IN NUTRITION

Description

Carbohydrates are polyhydroxy aldehydes, ketones, alcohols, acids, their simple derivatives and their polymers having linkages of the acetal type. They may be classified according to their degree of polymerization and may be divided initially into three principal groups, namely sugars, oligosaccharides and polysaccharides (see Figure 1).

Figure 1

The major dietary carbohydrates

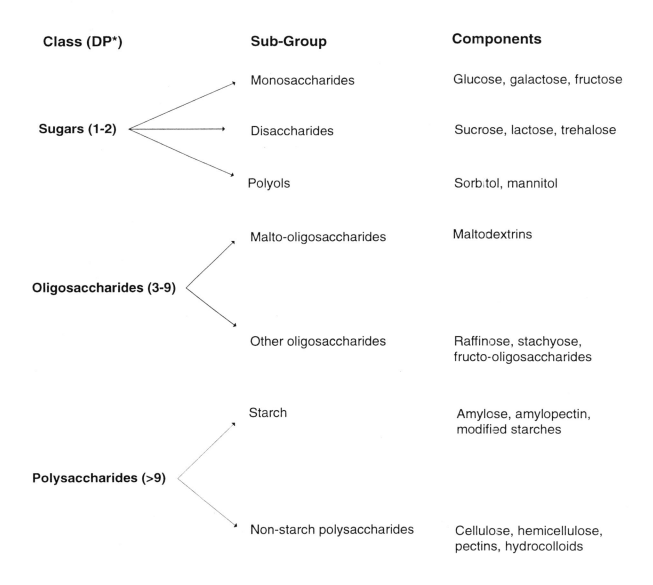

Class (DP*)	Sub-Group	Components
Sugars (1-2)	Monosaccharides	Glucose, galactose, fructose
	Disaccharides	Sucrose, lactose, trehalose
	Polyols	Sorbitol, mannitol
Oligosaccharides (3-9)	Malto-oligosaccharides	Maltodextrins
	Other oligosaccharides	Raffinose, stachyose, fructo-oligosaccharides
Polysaccharides (>9)	Starch	Amylose, amylopectin, modified starches
	Non-starch polysaccharides	Cellulose, hemicellulose, pectins, hydrocolloids

DP* = Degree of polymerization

Each of these three groups may be subdivided on the basis of the monosaccharide composition of the individual carbohydrates. Sugars comprise monosaccharides, disaccharides and polyols (sugar alcohols); oligosaccharides include malto-oligosaccharides, principally those occurring from the hydrolysis of starch, and other oligosaccharides, e.g. α-galactosides (raffinose, stachyose etc.) and fructo-oligosaccharides; the final group are the polysaccharides which may be divided into starch (α-glucans) and non-starch polysaccharides of which the major components are the polysaccharides of the plant cell wall such as cellulose, hemicellulose and pectin (2,3,4).

Total carbohydrate

Although the individual components of dietary carbohydrate are readily identifiable, there is some confusion as to what comprises total carbohydrate as reported in food tables. Two principal measures of total carbohydrate are used, firstly, that derived by "difference" and secondly the direct measurement of the individual components which are then combined to give a total. Calculating carbohydrates by "difference" has been used since the turn of the century. The protein, fat, ash and moisture content of a food are determined, subtracted from the total weight of the food and the remainder, or "difference", is considered to be carbohydrate. There are, however, a number of problems with this approach to total carbohydrate analysis in that the "by difference" figure includes a number of non-carbohydrate components such as lignin, organic acids, tannins, waxes, and some Maillard products. In addition to this error, it combines all of the analytical errors from the other analyses. Finally, a single global figure for carbohydrates in food is uninformative because it fails to identify the many types of carbohydrates in a food and thus to allow some understanding of the potential physiological properties of those carbohydrates (5,6).

Terminology

In deciding how to classify dietary carbohydrate the principal problem is to reconcile the various chemical divisions of carbohydrate with that which reflects physiology and health. A classification based purely on chemistry does not allow a ready translation into nutritional terms since each of the major classes of carbohydrate have a variety of physiological effects. However, a classification based on physiological properties also creates a number of problems in that it requires a single effect to be considered as overridingly important and to be used as the basis of the classification. This dichotomy has led to the introduction of a number of terms to describe various fractions and sub-fractions of carbohydrate (4,7).

Sugars

The term "sugars" is conventionally used to describe the mono and disaccharides. "Sugar", by contrast, is used to describe purified sucrose as are the terms "refined sugar" and "added sugar"

Extrinsic and intrinsic sugars

These terms had their origin in a United Kingdom (UK) Department of Health committee in 1989 (8), which was looking at the question of sugars in the diet. The terms were developed to help the consumer choose between what were considered to be healthy sugars and those which were not. Intrinsic sugars were defined as sugars occurring within the cell walls of plants, i.e. naturally occurring, while extrinsic sugars were those which were usually added to foods. Because lactose in milk is also an extrinsic sugar, an additional phrase "non-milk extrinsic sugars" was developed. These terms have not gained wide acceptance either in the UK or other countries in the world. There are no current plans to measure these sugars separately in the diet nor to incorporate their use into food tables.

Complex carbohydrates

This term was first used in the McGovern report, "Dietary Goals for the United States" in 1977 (9). The term was coined largely to distinguish sugars from other carbohydrates and in the report denotes "fruit, vegetables and whole-grains". The term has since come to be used to describe either starch alone, or the combination of all polysaccharides. It was used to encourage consumption of what were considered to be healthy foods such as whole-grain cereals, etc., but becomes meaningless when used to describe fruit and vegetables which are low in starch. Furthermore, it is now realized that starch, which is by any definition a complex carbohydrate, is variable metabolically with some forms being rapidly absorbed and having a high glycemic index and some being resistant to digestion. The term "complex carbohydrate" has encompassed, at various times, starch, dietary fibre and non-digestible oligosaccharides. As a substitute term for starch, however, it would seem to have little merit and, in principle, it is better to discuss carbohydrate components by using their common chemical names.

Available and unavailable carbohydrate

A major step forward conceptually in our understanding of carbohydrates was made by McCance and Lawrence in 1929 (10) with the division of dietary carbohydrate into available and unavailable. In an attempt to prepare food tables for diabetic diets they realised that not all carbohydrates could be "utilized and metabolized", i.e. provide the body with "carbohydrates for metabolism". Available carbohydrate was defined as "starch and soluble sugars" and unavailable as "mainly hemicellulose and fibre (cellulose)". This concept proved useful, not the least because it drew attention to the fact that some carbohydrate is not digested and absorbed in the small intestine but rather reaches the large bowel where it is fermented. It suggests that the site of digestion or fermentation in the gut of carbohydrate is of overriding importance. However, it is misleading to talk of carbohydrate as "unavailable" because some indigestible carbohydrate is able to provide the body with energy through fermentation. There are many properties of carbohydrate of which digestibility and fermentability are only two. A more appropriate substitute for the terms "available" and "unavailable" today would be to describe carbohydrates as either as glycemic (i.e. providing carbohydrate for metabolism) or non-glycemic, which is closer to the original concept of McCance and Lawrence.

Resistant starch

One of the major developments in our understanding of the importance of carbohydrates for health in the past twenty years has been the discovery of resistant starch. Resistant starch is defined as "starch and starch degradation products not absorbed in the small intestine of healthy humans" (11). The main forms of resistant starch are physically enclosed starch, e.g. within intact cell structures (RS_1), some raw starch granules (RS_2) and retrograded amylose (RS_3) (11,12).

Modified starch

The proportions of amylose and amylopectin in a starchy food is variable and can be altered by plant breeding. Techniques using genetic engineering are rapidly emerging, enabling starches to be produced for specific purposes by genetically modifying the crop used for their production. High amylose corn starch and high amylopectin (waxy) corn starch have been available for a long time, and display quite different functional as well as nutritional properties. High amylose starches require higher temperatures for gelatinization and are more prone to retrograde and to form amylose-lipid complexes. Such properties can be utilized in the formulation of foods with low glycemic index and/or high resistant starch content.

Physical modifications of starches include pregelatinization and partial hydrolysis (dextrinization). Chemical modification is mainly the introduction of side groups and cross-linking or oxidation. These modifications may be used to decrease viscosity and to improve gel stability, mouthfeel, appearance and texture, and resistance for heat treatment (13). The application of modified starches as fat replacers is another important area. Some modified starches may be partly resistant to digestion in the small intestine, thereby adding to resistant starch (14).

Dietary fibre

The original description of dietary fibre by Trowell in 1972 (15) was "that portion of food which is derived from cellular walls of plants which is digested very poorly by human beings". This is not an exact description of any carbohydrate in the diet but is more a physiological concept. It was linked by Burkitt and Trowell to the etiology of a number of "Western diseases" (16) and on the basis of this a hypothesis relating fibre to health was developed. The use of the term has, however, caused many difficulties over the years because of controversies regarding definition. Moreover, the proposal that there are a number of dietary fibre deficiency disorders is an over-simplification and needs to be modified now in the light of new knowledge of diet and disease.

The main components of dietary fibre are derived from the cell walls of plant material in the diet and comprise cellulose, hemicellulose and pectin (the non-starch polysaccharides). Lignin, a non-carbohydrate component of the cell wall is also often included. Dietary fibre is a term which is felt to be valuable for the consumer who looks upon this as a healthy component of the diet. At the present time there is no consensus as to which components of carbohydrate should be included as dietary fibre and different authors have variously included non-starch polysaccharides and resistant starch. More recently it has been suggested that non-digestible oligosaccharides should also be included. Dietary fibre has also been defined by method. While there is general agreement that the non-starch polysaccharides are the principal part of dietary fibre there is currently no consensus as to whether other components should be included in this term. It has been suggested that the use of the term dietary fibre be gradually phased out (1,17). Its widespread use and popularity with the consumer has made this difficult in practice and the term has been useful in nutrition education and product development.

Soluble and insoluble fibre

These terms developed out of the early chemistry of non-starch polysaccharides which showed that the fractional extraction of these polysaccharides could be controlled by changing the pH of solutions. They proved very useful in the initial understanding of the physiological properties of dietary fibre, allowing a simple division into those which principally had effects on glucose and lipid absorption from the small intestine (soluble) and those which were slowly and incompletely fermented and had more pronounced effects on bowel habit (insoluble). However, the separation of soluble and insoluble fractions is not chemically very distinct being dependent on the conditions of extraction (18). Moreover, the physiological differences are not, in fact, so distinct with much insoluble fibre being rapidly and completely fermented while not all soluble fibre has effects on glucose and lipid absorption.

Methodology for dietary carbohydrate analysis

Mono- and disaccharides

They can be analyzed specifically by enzymatic, gas-liquid chromatography (GLC) or high performance liquid chromatography (HPLC) methods. Depending on the food matrix to be analyzed, extraction of the low molecular weight carbohydrates in aqueous ethanol, usually 80% (v/v), may be advisable before analysis (5,6,7).

The enzymatic procedures are based on specific, highly purified enzymes and have been instrumental in providing means of specific and precise analysis of individual carbohydrates in mixtures without a large investment in instrumentation. Enzymatic methods are still preferable when one single carbohydrate is to be analyzed, e.g. glucose, as the end point of starch analysis.

When several different monosaccharides are to be determined simultaneously, HPLC or GLC methods are preferable. HPLC systems using sensitive amperometric detectors are gaining in popularity over GLC, in that the derivatization necessary before the GLC determination is avoided.

Polyols

Polyols are usually determined by GLC using alditol acetate derivatives. HPLC methods are also available.

Oligosaccharides

Oligosaccharides can also be determined by GLC or HPLC methods. These methods work well for purified preparations, but in complex foods or diets, enzymatic hydrolysis and determination of liberated monosaccharides is an alternative for specific determination. Malto-oligosaccharides are recovered as "starch" if not extracted before starch analysis.

Separation of oligosaccharides from polysaccharides

By definition, polysaccharides have 10 or more monomeric units, and oligosaccharides less than 10. Analytically, separation is based on solubility in aqueous ethanol, usually around 80% (v/v). The alcohol solubility of carbohydrates, however, is dependent not only on the degree of polymerization (DP), but also on the molecular structure. For instance, highly branched carbohydrates may be soluble in 80% ethanol in spite of a DP considerably higher than 10. In practice, therefore, the separation of oligosaccharides from polysaccharides is empirical and does not provide an exact division based on DP (18).

Starch

Quantitative analysis of starch in foods by most current methods is based on enzymatic degradation and specific determination of liberated glucose. Nutritionally, starch can be divided into glucogenic ("available") and resistant starch, which is not absorbed in the small intestine. Resistant starch is poorly soluble in water and methods aiming at a total starch analysis employ an initial 2M potassium hydroxide (KOH) or dimethylsulfoxide solvent (DMSO) treatment to disperse crystalline starch fractions that would otherwise remain unhydrolyzed. Methods for measuring resistant starch are still in their infancy and have not yet been tested in formal collaborative studies. They aim at simulating normal starch digestion in the small intestine. A key step is to mimic the normal disintegration of the food which occurs during chewing. One method uses a standardized milling/homogenization technique (12), whereas others employ standardized chewing by volunteers (19,20). Both approaches have been evaluated against human ileostomy experiments with a limited number of food matrices (21).

Non-starch polysaccharides (NSP)

The determination of NSP is based on the following steps: (a) degradation of starch by enzymatic hydrolysis after solublization, (b) removal of low molecular weight carbohydrates, including starch hydrolysis products, (c) hydrolysis of the NSP to their constituent monomers, and (d) quantitative determination of those monomers. The acid hydrolysis step is a critical one, and it has to be designed as an optimal balance between complete hydrolysis and destruction of the liberated monomers (22,23).

The most widely-used method today for specific determination of the liberated monomers is GLC with alditol acetate derivatives. HPLC detection is an alternative gaining in popularity. Colourimetric determination is still preferred for uronic acids, which are derived mainly from pectic substances. A colourimetric method is also available for total NSP.

Fractions of NSP, such as cellulose and non-cellulosic polysaccharides, can be separated by using sequential extraction and hydrolysis methods. For instance, cellulose is not hydrolysed by dilute (1-2M) sulphuric acid, unless it has first been dispersed in concentrated acid.

Dietary fibre

Three methods for dietary fibre analysis have undergone extensive testing in recent years, including collaborative studies satisfactory enough for official approval of bodies such as the AOAC International (Association of Official Analytical Chemists) and the Bureau Communautaire de Référence (BCR) of the European Community (24):

1. The enzymatic, gravimetric AOAC methods of Prosky and co-workers, and subsequently Lee and co-workers.

2. The enzymatic-chemical methods of Englyst and co-workers.

3. The enzymatic-chemical method of Theander and co-workers (the Uppsala method).

The enzymatic-gravimetric AOAC methods are derived from methods aiming at simulating the digestion in the human small intestine to isolate an undigested residue as a measure of dietary fibre. This residue is corrected for associated ash and protein. Since no DMSO or KOH dispersion is used, starch that resists the amylases used in the assay will remain as a fibre component. Since the sample has to be milled, and since a heat-stable amylase (termamyl) is used at a temperature close to $100^{\circ}C$, physically enclosed starch (RS_1) and resistant starch granules (RS_2) will not be included. Retrograded amylose (RS_3) that is included is the main form of resistant starch (RS) in processed foods. Lignin, a non-carbohydrate component of the dietary fibre complex is also included, as well as some tannins. These components are a very small proportion of most foods but can be substantial in some unconventional raw materials or special "fibre" preparations (25).

The Englyst method measures the NSP specifically, either as individual monomeric components by GLC (or HPLC) or colourimetrically as reducing substances (total NSP) . Accordingly, DMSO is used initially to ensure a complete removal of starch, and lignin is not determined. The difference between estimates with the gravimetric methods and the Englyst method is mainly due to resistant starch and lignin (24).

The Uppsala method employs hydrolysis conditions and GLC determination of monomers in a similar way as in the Englyst method. However, DMSO is not employed for starch dispersion, and a gravimetric estimate of lignin (Klason lignin) is added to obtain the dietary fibre. The Uppsala method and the gravimetric AOAC methods give very concordant results (24).

Labelling

Food labelling has two main aims: to inform the consumer of the composition of the food and to assist them in the selection of a healthy diet. These two aims are not always easy to reconcile because the health benefit of different carbohydrate-containing foods cannot readily be communicated simply from a description of their composition.

Labelling should be based on the chemical classification used in Figure 1. Analytical methods should be clearly defined and validated. The principal information should be total carbohydrate, measured as the sum of the individual components. Further information on carbohydrate composition, based on the classification in Figure 1, could include terms such as sugars, starch and non-starch polysaccharides. Other terms, such as non-digestible oligosaccharides (NDO), polyols, resistant starch and dietary fibre may be used, provided the components included in these terms are clearly defined.

Availability and consumption

Trends in the supply and intake of carbohydrates can be studied by four principal approaches:

1.   Production
2.   Food balance sheets
3.   Household surveys
4.   Individual assessments

Food production statistics, which are available from FAO for every country in the world and for every crop, are useful for examining trends in consumption (26). From these data it can be seen that the major sources of carbohydrate in the human diet are:

1.   Cereals
2.   Root crops
3.   Sugar crops
4.   Pulses
5.   Vegetables
6.   Fruit
7.   Milk products

Sustainability

Trends over the last 20-30 years indicate growth in world production of cereals, sugar cane, vegetables and fruit. On the other hand, production of root crops, pulses and sugar beet has changed little on a world basis. Marked decreases have actually been seen in pulse production in some countries in Asia, and in root crop production in Europe. This suggests a change in food preference away from roots and pulses and towards cereals. Examination of eating habits in a number of countries indicates that this is the case (27-29). Since root crops are an excellent source of carbohydrate, there is concern about this downward trend in production.

Populations continue to grow in most parts of the world and, overall, food production would seem to be keeping pace with population growth. Increased production is due to improved agricultural practices rather than increased crop area, the major reason for increases being greater use of fertilizer (30-32). There are, however, specific countries where this is not happening. For the entire continent of Africa, cereal production is inadequate.

A major question is how much more improvement and efficiency in production can be achieved, and whether the amount of carbohydrate will be sufficient for the world's population in the future. Projections for future growth suggest problems ahead, particularly in Africa (33).

Changing patterns of consumption

Both food balance information and results from individual assessments are used to determine carbohydrate intakes. Food balance data is intended to describe food available for consumption. It is unlikely to do so because it does not include home production, which is variable from country to country, and may be considerable in some developing countries (34,35). As a reflection of food consumed, food balance data is questionable, since it does not include food wasted or spoiled, or used for purposes other than human food, the proportion of which may change from year to year. As a result, food balance data for individual countries has failed to demonstrate the changes in consumption of carbohydrates which are seen using individual surveys (36-38).

Data from individual surveys also have limitations. Surveys are carried out by a variety of methodologies. While each has advantages and disadvantages, all suffer from a degree of underreporting. This can be intentional or involuntary, most likely due to individuals forgetting food items or not describing foods thought to be undesirable (35). There is also the failure to record data or the altering of actual diets. The difference, then, between food balance data and individual assessments, for energy and nutrient intakes, is not only the form of wastage and spoilage on the food balance side of the equation, but also the underreporting on the individual intake side. True food intakes therefore lie somewhere between food balance and individual intake estimates (35). Another major problem is the varied carbohydrate terminology used in different countries. Many countries express total carbohydrate 'by difference', rather than as carbohydrate analyzed directly, and this results in overestimates of the percent energy derived from carbohydrate. There is also a great variety in terms used to describe simple sugars, such as "sugars", "sugar", "refined sugar", "added sugar", "sucrose", and "sugars minus lactose". Often there is no description of what is being reported (39). There is a need to standardize the terminology for carbohydrate and its components in individual surveys and a need for consistency in both reporting and the description of the terms used.

In spite of terminology difficulties, it is possible to gain a picture of carbohydrate intakes and trends. Annex 1 gives the intakes of carbohydrate and components where available, from a number of surveys since 1980. As a percent of energy, total carbohydrate ranges from about 40% to over 80%, with the developed countries, such as those in North America, Western Europe and Australia at the low end of the range, and developing countries in Asia and Africa at the high end. Starch accounts for 20%-50% or more of energy where the total carbohydrate intake is in the high range. Sugars account for 9%-27% of energy intake; where total carbohydrate is high, sugar intake is generally low. Where data are available, intake of carbohydrate as a percent of energy is higher for children than for adults.

Trends in consumption indicate a falling carbohydrate intake in developed countries until the last two decades (39). During that time some increase has been noted as fat intakes fall. The major sources of carbohydrate are cereals, representing over 50% of all carbohydrate consumed in both developed and developing countries, with sugar crops the next major source, followed by root crops, fruits, vegetables, pulses and milk products. In some of the developing countries much of the carbohydrate is derived from a single food source such as rice, cassava or maize. Carbohydrate foods are an important vehicle for protein, micronutrients and other food components, like phytochemicals, which have important benefits for health. Individual food sources vary, however, in the provision of these components. A single food source of carbohydrate is therefore undesirable and populations whose diets are primarily based on a single food can suffer from micronutrient deficiencies due to lack of variety. It is important, therefore, that a number of different carbohydrate sources be consumed and efforts should be made to encourage a wide variety of carbohydrate foods.

Data on intake of sources of sugars is only available for developed countries. These data show similar proportions of sugars are derived from cereal products, milk products and beverages, among these countries. There is some variation in the proportions derived from fruit and confectionery, with the UK consuming less fruit and higher amounts of confectionery than countries such as the United States and Australia (40-44).

Intakes of non-starch polysaccharides (45) range from about 19g/day in some countries in Europe and North America, to nearly 30g/day in rural Africa (46-48). Cereals are again the major source of this component. Data on intake of dietary fibre, determined by methods such as that of the AOAC (Association of Official Analytical Chemists) (49) and the older Southgate method (50), are about 15-20 g/day for North America, Europe and Australia, to 25-40 g/day for countries in Asia and Africa (47, 51-53).

Physiology

Carbohydrates have a wide range of physiological effects which may be important to health, such as:

- Provision of energy
- Effects on satiety/gastric emptying
- Control of blood glucose and insulin metabolism
- Protein glycosylation
- Cholesterol and triglyceride metabolism
- Bile acid dehydroxylation
- Fermentation-   Hydrogen/methane production
                          Short-chain fatty acids production
                          Control of colonic epithelial cell function
- Bowel habit/laxation/motor activity
- Effects on large bowel microflora

Carbohydrate as an energy source

Dietary carbohydrates have by convention been given an energy value of 4 kcal/g (17 kJ/g), although where carbohydrates are expressed as monosaccharides, the value of 3.75 kcal/g (15.7 kJ/g) is used. It is now clear, however, that a number of carbohydrates are only partly or not at all digested in the small intestine and are fermented in the large bowel to short chain fatty acids. These include the non-digestible oligosaccharides, resistant starch and non-starch polysaccharides. The process of fermentation is metabolically less efficient than absorption in the small intestine and these carbohydrates provide the body with less energy.

In light of a new understanding of the digestion and metabolism of carbohydrate and developments in methodology, the energy value of all carbohydrates in the diet should be reassessed and more accurate energy factors assigned to each group or sub-group. There are a number of potential approaches to accomplish this. These include the classic calorimetry experiments similar to those first undertaken by Atwater, as well as human balance studies and ileostomy recovery experiments. Knowledge of the chemistry of individual carbohydrates allows a prediction to be made regarding their digestion or fermentation, and an energy value to be assigned. *In vitro* models of fermentation can be constructed and from these the fermentation stoichiometry can be deduced. Studies using stable isotope tracer techniques may also be of value.

While the energy yield of carbohydrate delivered to the colon will vary according to the extent of colonic fermentation (or the assumptions made in the model used), there may be an argument for assigning a single energy value to all such carbohydrate. Published studies suggest that a caloric value of about 2 kcal/g (8 kJ/g) (54,55) would be a reasonable average figure for carbohydrate which reaches the colon. While individual carbohydrates will have different values, in the range of 1-2 kcal/g, these differences are unlikely to be of importance to health.

Satiety

The possibility of controlling hunger, satiety and food intake by altering the type of carbohydrate in food has intrigued a number of investigators (56). At present the variability of the findings and the lack of understanding of a clear relationship to physiologic parameters thought to be involved in the regulation of food intake limit practical application of this approach. It is unlikely that controlling a single dietary component, such as the type of sugar or starch, will lead to significant changes in the amount of food consumed. Also, compensation for small dietary changes made in one meal may often be seen at a subsequent meal. A better approach to controlling hunger and increasing satiety is likely to be associated with changes in the composition of the total diet (57).

Glucose and insulin

The digestion of dietary carbohydrates starts in the mouth, where salivary α-amylase initiates starch degradation. The starch fragments thus formed include maltose, some glucose and dextrins containing the 1,6-α-glycosidic branching points of amylopectin. The α-amylase degradation of starch is completed by the pancreatic amylase active in the small intestine.

Dietary disaccharides, as well as degradation products of starch, need to be broken down to monosaccharides in order to be absorbed. This final hydrolysis is accomplished by hydrolases attached to the intestinal brush-border membrane, referred to as "disaccharidases". Disaccharidase deficiencies occur as rare genetic defects, causing malabsorption and intolerance of the corresponding disaccharide.

Glucose and galactose are transported actively against a concentration gradient into the intestinal mucosal cells by a sodium dependent transporter (SGLT 1). Fructose undergoes facilitated transport by another mechanism (GLUT 5). Fructose taken together with other sugars (as in naturally fructose-containing foods) is better absorbed than fructose alone (58).

When delivered to the circulation, the absorbed carbohydrates cause an elevation of the blood glucose concentration. Fructose and galactose have to be converted to glucose mainly in the liver and therefore produce less pronounced blood glucose elevation. The extent and duration of the blood glucose rise after a meal is dependent upon the rate of absorption, which in turn depends upon factors such as gastric emptying as well as the rate of hydrolysis and diffusion of hydrolysis products in the small intestine.

Insulin is secreted as a response to blood glucose elevation but is modified by many neural and endocrine stimuli. Insulin secretion is also influenced by food related factors, especially by the amount and the amino acid composition of dietary proteins. Insulin has important regulatory functions in both carbohydrate and lipid metabolism and is necessary for glucose uptake by most body cells.

Lactose

Lactose, a β-linked disaccharide of glucose and galactose, is the principal sugar in milk. At birth, lactase activity is high in the brush-border of the small bowel of infants, but declines after weaning so that most populations of the world have low activity in adult life. The exceptions are Caucasian peoples and some other population groups in whom the majority retain a high lactase activity throughout life (59,60).

During the years since 1980, there has been a major change in the way lactose absorption is viewed and a resultant shift away from the concept that lactose "malabsorption" is a pathological state. Low mucosal lactase activity in adults is the norm throughout most of the world. However, such a state usually allows the drinking of modest quantities of milk spaced throughout the day without adverse symptoms. Milk consumption is therefore now being encouraged in many areas of the world because of its value as a source of protein, calcium and riboflavin. Fermented milk products, which have lower lactose content and contain enzymes and microorganisms that can assist in lactose digestion, are better tolerated than milk. Technology exists to reduce the lactose level in foods and this should be taken into consideration when milk is included as food aid. Cheese, however, has almost no lactose.

Lactose which is not digested, passes into the colon where it is fermented. In some individuals this causes lactose intolerance, the term used to describe the clinical symptoms of abdominal discomfort, flatulence and diarrhoea, associated with the ingestion of lactose containing foods by persons with low lactase activity. It also occurs as a transient phenomenon when the intestinal mucosa is injured following acute infection in children and in protein-energy malnutrition. It is also found in adults, particularly in association with coeliac disease and tropical sprue. In these conditions, lactose malabsorption is said to be "secondary" to intestinal mucosal disease. A small proportion of the Caucasian population also exhibits low lactase activity and lactose intolerance.

Protein glycosylation

The non-enzymatic glycation of proteins is dependent on the concentration of glucose and fructose in blood and the half-life of the protein. The initial reaction is between the monosaccharide and the amino group of an amino acid, usually lysine, to form a Shiff base which undergoes rearrangement and formation of Amadori products. As the reaction progresses, increasingly complex Maillard products are formed with the eventual production of Advanced Glycation End-products or AGEs which are associated with irreversible loss of protein function. The extent of glycation of specific proteins, such as Haemoglobin A1c in diabetics serves as an indication of medium term control of blood glucose. Examples of functional changes induced by glycation include lens proteins in the eye with resultant cataract formation, increased microvascular complications, abnormal fibrin network formation and impaired fibrinolysis. These changes are most clearly seen in diabetic patients (61,62).

Lipids and bile acids

There has been concern that a substantial increase in carbohydrate-containing food at the expense of fat, might result in a decrease in high-density lipoprotein and a corresponding increase in very low-density lipoprotein and triglycerides in the blood. However, there is no evidence that this happens when the increase in carbohydrates occurs as a result of increased consumption of vegetables, fruits and appropriately processed cereals over prolonged periods.

Polysaccharides like oat β-glucan, guar gum and those from psyllium have been repeatedly shown to lower serum cholesterol levels in those with elevated levels, with little change if serum levels are normal (63,64). Proposed mechanisms include impaired bile acid and cholesterol reabsorption through physical entrapment in the small intestine, or inhibitory effects on cholesterol synthesis by products of lower bowel fermentation, particularly propionic acid. Not all fermentable polysaccharides are effective, however, and recent studies have indicated that neither oligosaccharides nor resistant starch have a significant effect on serum lipids in young normolipidemic subjects (21,65).

Fermentation

Fermentation is the colonic phase of the digestive process and describes the breakdown in the large intestine of carbohydrates not digested and absorbed in the upper gut. This process involves gut microflora and is unique to the colon of humans because it occurs without the availability of oxygen. It thus results in the formation of the gases hydrogen, methane and carbon dioxide, as well as short chain fatty acids (SCFA) (acetate, propionate and butyrate), and stimulates bacterial growth (biomass). The gases are either absorbed and excreted in breath, or passed out via the rectum. The major products of such fermentation are the SCFA which are rapidly absorbed and metabolized by the body. Acetate passes primarily into the blood and is taken up by liver, muscle and other tissues. Propionate is a major glucose precursor in ruminant animals such as the cow and sheep, but this is not an important pathway in humans. Butyrate is metabolized primarily by colonocytes and has been shown to regulate cell growth, and to induce differentiation and apoptosis (66).

Bowel habit

It has long been known that non-starch polysaccharides are the principal dietary component affecting laxation. This occurs through increases in bowel content bulk and a speeding up of intestinal transit time. The extent of the effect depends on the chemical and physical nature of the polysaccharides and the extent to which they are fermented in the colon. Fermentable polysaccharides stimulate increases in microbial biomass in the colon, resulting in some increase in fecal weight, but not to the extent of non-fermentable polysaccharides. The latter are not significantly degraded in the colon and become consituents of the stool. In so doing, they hold water and produce a marked increase in fecal weight. Similarly, resistant starch can increase fecal weight, but this again depends on the extent of fermentation (67).

Microflora

Carbohydrate which is fermented stimulates the growth of bacteria in the large gut. This is a generalized effect which leads to an increase in the total number of bacteria or biomass. When bacterial growth occurs, the microflora synthesize protein actively from preformed amino acids and peptides as well as some de-novo synthesis using ammonia as the source of nitrogen. The additional biomass is excreted in feces and is one of the mechanisms whereby carbohydrate influences bowel habit. The increased biomass excretion is accompanied by increased nitrogen excretion. The efficiency of conversion of carbohydrate to biomass is determined principally by the type of substrate, the rate of breakdown and the transit time through the large intestine (68).

One of the more significant developments in recent years with regard to the gut microflora has been the demonstration that specific dietary carbohydrates selectively stimulate the growth of individual groups or species of bacteria. An example of this is the effect of fructo-oligosaccharides on the growth of bifidobacteria. The importance of bifidobacteria is that they may be one of the major contributors to colonization resistance in the colon, thereby protecting the host from invasion by pathogenic species. Foods which selectively stimulate the growth of gut bacteria are known as pre-biotics (69).

CHAPTER 2
THE ROLE OF CARBOHYDRATES IN MAINTENANCE OF HEALTH

Carbohydrates in the diet

While the amount of carbohydrate required to avoid ketosis is very small (about 50 g/day), carbohydrate provides the majority of energy in the diets of most people. There are many reasons why this is desirable. In addition to providing easily available energy for oxidative metabolism, carbohydrate-containing foods are vehicles for important micronutrients and phytochemicals. Dietary carbohydrate is important to maintain glycemic homeostasis and for gastrointestinal integrity and function. Unlike fat and protein, high levels of dietary carbohydrate, provided it is obtained from a variety of sources, is not associated with adverse health effects. Finally, diets high in carbohydrate as compared to those high in fat, reduce the likelihood of developing obesity and its co-morbid conditions. An optimum diet should consist of at least 55% of total energy coming from carbohydrate obtained from a variety of food sources.

The consultation agreed that when carbohydrate consumption levels are at or above 75% of total energy there could be significant adverse effects on nutritional status by the exclusion of adequate quantities of protein, fat and other essential nutrients. In arriving at its recommendation of a minimum of 55% of total energy from carbohydrate, the consultation realised that a significant percentage of total energy needs to be provided by protein and fat, but that their contribution to total energy intakes will vary from one country to another on the basis of food consumption patterns and food availability.

Energy balance

In adults, it is important that the amount of energy ingested be matched to the amount of energy expended. Maintenance of energy balance is important in order to avoid obesity and its associated co-morbidities such as diabetes and cardiovascular disease. Positive energy balance and obesity occur when total energy intake exceeds total energy expenditure, regardless of composition of the excess energy. However, the composition of the diet can affect whether and to what extent positive energy balance occurs.

The composition of the diet can also affect the ability to maintain energy balance. In particular, diets containing at least 55% of energy from a variety of carbohydrate sources, as compared to high fat diets, reduce the likelihood that body fat accumulation will occur. Substantial data suggest that diets high in fat content tend to promote consumption of more total energy than diets high in carbohydrates (58,70). This effect may be due to the low energy density of high carbohydrate diets, since total volume of food consumed appears to provide an important satiety cue (71). There are no data to suggest that different types of carbohydrates differentially affect total energy intake.

In addition to affecting the chance of having excess energy available, the composition of the diet also affects the proportion of excess energy that will be stored as body fat. The body has a large fat storage capacity and excess dietary fat is stored very efficiently in adipose tissue. Alternatively, the body's capacity to store carbohydrate is limited and excess carbohydrate is not efficiently stored as body fat (72). Instead, excess carbohydrate tends to be oxidized, leading to indirect fat accumulation via reductions in fat oxidation (73).

Excess fat and carbohydrate were previously thought to be equally fattening. This was due to the assumption that *de novo* lipogenesis was a commonly used pathway for disposal of excess carbohydrate. The available data suggest, however, that this process occurs rarely in human subjects and only in situations of appreciable carbohydrate overfeeding (74). In most usual circumstances, accumulation of body fat via *de novo* lipogenesis is quantitatively very low.

While noting the low overall contribution of *de novo* lipogensis to body fat accumulation, it should be noted that *de novo* lipogenesis is increased with insulin resistance and with extremely high consumption of sucrose or fructose (74).

Physical activity

Maintenance of energy balance is dependent both on energy intake and energy expenditure. Maintaining regular physical activity greatly reduces the likelihood of creating positive energy balance, regardless of the composition of the diet. There is agreement that the combination of a high carbohydrate diet and regular physical activity is the optimal arrangement to avoid positive energy balance and obesity.

The increased energy needs of physical activity can be supplied by carbohydrate or fat. The importance of carbohydrate in the diet becomes more critical as the amount and intensity of physical activity increases.

In many developing countries, the major challenge is to meet daily energy needs created by high levels of daily physical labour. In such cases, any combination of carbohydrate and fat which provides sufficient energy is to be encouraged.

Many countries recommend increasing leisure time physical activity. While increased physical activity would clearly increase energy needs, these do not create needs for specific macronutrients. Rather, the optimum diet identified above is considered sufficient to provide for such physical activity.

There is substantial evidence that supplemental carbohydrate can improve performance for the elite endurance-trained athlete. A high carbohydrate diet during a few days preceding an endurance event, carbohydrate loading, a high carbohydrate pre-event meal and carbohydrate supplementation in the form of carbohydrate-containing beverages have all been shown to enhance performance during long-distance cycling and running. There is, however, no evidence that such carbohydrate supplementation would improve perfomance for the majority of people who engage in recreational physical activity of lower intensity and duration. On the other hand, carbohydrate intake following exercise can help to quickly replenish depleted glycogen stores (75).

Carbohydrate and behaviour

It has been suggested that food intake could have important effects on behaviour. While providing breakfast to children who do not typically eat breakfast can increase cognitive performance (76), it is less clear that the overall composition of the diet can affect behaviour. It has been suggested that sugar consumption leads to hyperactivity in children. However, an extensive review of the literature in this area (77) concluded that there is no evidence to support the claim that refined sugar intake has any significant influence on either behaviour or cognitive performance in children.

Because glucose is an essential fuel for the central nervous system, carbohydrate has also been suggested to play a role in memory and cognitive function. While there appears to be a relationship between glucose levels and memory processing, the clinical significance of this relationship remains unclear.

Carbohydrate through the life cycle

Energy and nutrient needs are increased in pregnancy and lactation, and the primary challenge for pregnant women is to meet these increased energy needs in order to ensure healthy offspring. It has been observed that where variety in the food supply is low and carbohydrate intake is high, a low birth weight is more common. This raises concerns about the adequacy of high carbohydrate diets to meet the energy and nutrient needs of pregnancy when food variety is limited. Energy and nutrient needs should be met by consumption of a wide variety of carbohydrate foods. There is also some concern about excessive fat intake in pregnancy since it may be associated with risk of obesity in the mother.

In many countries, infants receive 45-55% of energy from fat through breastmilk or formulas and 35-45% of energy from carbohydrate. While specific reductions in fat intake are not recommended below the age of two years, infants in many countries consume lower fat diets. This does not present a problem as long as energy requirements are fulfilled. From the age of two and on, the optimum diet (at least 55% of total energy from a variety of carbohydrate sources) should be gradually introduced.

During the first four to six months of life, exclusive breast feeding is recommended as this tailors the concentration of lactose to the maturing neonatal and infant gut, particularly while colonic microflora and pancreatic amylase production are developing. For infants fed on formula, the carbohydrate and other nutrient components should usually mimic breast milk to the extent possible and in accordance with standards of the Codex Alimentarius (78).

Carbohydrate digestion in the neonate and young infant is significantly influenced by both gastrointestinal maturation and the chemical nature of the carbohydrate ingested. The establishment of colonic microflora is responsible for colonic carbohydrate scavenging, converting any carbohydrate entering the colon into short chain fatty acids. Any disturbances or inappropriate development of this microflora (incorrect infant formula, antibiotics, infection) leads to colonic carbohydrate overloading and diarrhoea.

Lactose from dairy products can be a major source of carbohydrate for young children. In addition, milk represents an excellent source of high quality protein, calcium, and riboflavin. In most populations, even those with low lactase activity, milk can be ingested in small amounts, especially after meals with dilution by co-ingestion. Fermented dairy products can be valuable items in the diet of most people irrespective of intestinal lactase status.

Often the transition from childhood to adulthood is associated with changes in dietary pattern. In developing countries, children frequently consume very high carbohydrate intakes from a single or a small number of sources, while adults have greater variety. In such cases, the adult diet is preferred. In developed countries, on the other hand, surveys indicate that children have higher intakes of carbohydrate from more sources than adults. In those countries, the diet consumed by children would seem to be more beneficial. In both situations, at least 55% of carbohydrate energy from a variety of sources is the optimum.

Individualization of carbohydrate intake is necessary for elderly populations. Elderly individuals in many countries are at risk as regards both malnutrition and obesity. Food intake patterns can be altered by changes in taste perception, chronic disease and medication use. While a high carbohydrate diet is recommended for prevention of weight gain and obesity, it should be recognized that some individuals may need diets higher in energy density (e.g. fats) in order to prevent malnutrition. Optimizing intake of carbohydrate to minimize glucose intolerance in later life is a consideration in countries where such intolerance is a problem.

CHAPTER 3

DIETARY CARBOHYDRATE AND DISEASE

Carbohydrates may directly influence human diseases by affecting physiological and metabolic processes, thereby reducing risk factors for the disease or the disease process itself. Carbohydrates may also have indirect effects on diseases, for example, by displacing other nutrients or facilitating increased intakes of a wide range of other substances frequently found in carbohydrate-containing foods. Evidence of associations between carbohydrates and diseases comes from epidemiological and clinical studies. There are relatively few examples in which direct causal links between carbohydrates and diseases have been proven. Thus the nutrient-disease or food-disease associations discussed below must be considered in terms of the strength of evidence from a range of observational studies and clinical experiments and the existence of plausible hypotheses.

Obesity

The frequency of obesity has increased dramatically in many developed and developing countries. This is of profound public health importance because of the clearly defined negative effect of obesity, especially when centrally distributed, in relation to diabetes, coronary heart disease and other chronic diseases of lifestyle. Genetic and environmental factors play a role in determining the propensity for obesity in populations and individuals. Lack of physical activity is believed to contribute to the increasing rates of obesity observed in many countries and may be a factor in whether an individual who is at risk will become overweight or obese.

High carbohydrate foods promote satiety in the short term. As fat is stored more efficiently than excess carbohydrate, use of high carbohydrate foods is likely to reduce the risk of obesity in the long term. Much controversy surrounds the extent to which sugars and starch promote obesity. There is no direct evidence to implicate either of these groups of carbohydrates in the etiology of obesity, based on data derived from studies in affluent societies. Nevertheless, it is important to reiterate that excess energy in any form will promote body fat accumulation and that excess consumption of low fat foods, while not as obesity-producing as excess consumption of high fat products, will lead to obesity if energy expenditure is not increased. While high carbohydrate diets may help reduce the risk of obesity by preventing overconsumption of energy, there is no evidence to suggest that the macronutrient composition of a low energy diet influences the rate and extent of weight loss in the treatment of obese patients.

Non-insulin dependent diabetes mellitus (NIDDM)

High rates of NIDDM in all population groups are associated with rapid cultural changes in populations previously consuming traditional diets, and also with increasing obesity, especially when centrally distributed. Although the precise mode of inheritance has not been established, there is no doubt that genetic factors are involved. Certain populations appear to have a strong predisposition to the development of NIDDM to the extent that in some groups about half the adult population have the disease (79). Within all populations a family history of NIDDM is an important predisposing factor. Diet and lifestyle-related conditions which may lead to obesity will clearly influence the risk of developing NIDDM in populations and individuals who are susceptible to this condition. Foods rich in non-starch polysaccharides and carbohydrate-containing foods with a low glycemic index appear to protect against diabetes, the effect being independent of body mass index. In terms of disease prevention, it is not possible on the basis of current data to distinguish the relative merits of different types of non-starch polysaccharides. Some epidemiological evidence suggests particular benefit of appropriately processed cereal foods, while other epidemiological and clinical studies suggest benefits of non-starch polysaccharide from legumes and pectin-rich foods. Thus, avoiding obesity and increasing intakes of a wide range of foods rich in non-starch polysaccharide and carbohydrate-containing foods with a low glycemic index offers the best means of reducing the rapidly increasing rates of NIDDM in many countries.

Consuming a wide range of carbohydrate foods is now regarded as acceptable in the nutritional management of people who have already developed NIDDM. It has been suggested that between 60 and 70 per cent of total energy should be derived from a mix of mono-unsaturated fatty acids and carbohydrates. Carbohydrates should principally be derived from a wide range of appropriately processed cereals, vegetables and fruit, with particular emphasis on those foods which have a low glycemic index. The goal to achieve and maintain ideal body weight remains paramount, ensuring that foods high in fat which might predispose to obesity are not encouraged, even though they might have a low glycemic index.

Sucrose and other sugars have not been directly implicated in the etiology of diabetes and recommendations concerning intake relate primarily to the avoidance of all energy-dense foods in order to reduce obesity. Most recommendations for the management of diabetes permit modest (30-50 g/day) intakes of sucrose and other added sugars in the diabetic dietary prescription provided these are: a) consumed within the context of total energy allowance; b) nutrient-dense foods and foods rich in non-starch polysaccharides are not displaced; and, c) they are incorporated as part of a mixed meal. In some populations where fat intake is relatively low and sucrose intake high, a reduced intake of sucrose may be considered in the diabetic dietary prescription.

Increased meal frequency under iso-energetic conditions does not, in the long term, appear to be associated with any alteration in glycemic control. This suggests that personal preference is the key determinant of meal frequency, provided that body weight and daily (as well as long-term) glycemic control are not adversely influenced. Special diabetic food products are not generally recommended and fructose is not regarded as having any particular merits as a sweetener when compared with other added sugars. However, low-energy beverages containing alternative non-nutritive sweeteners may be useful for people with diabetes.

Dietary factors have not been conclusively shown to be risk factors for insulin-dependent diabetes and the key advice concerning carbohydrates in the management of this condition concerns distribution of intake of carbohydrates during the day. Carbohydrate intake needs to be regularly distributed and balanced with injected insulin. The general principles of the diabetic dietary approach to non-insulin dependent diabetes may also be applied to those with insulin-dependent diabetes.

Cardiovascular disease

Many genetic and lifestyle factors are involved in the etiology of coronary heart disease and influence both the atherosclerotic and thrombotic processes underlying the clinical manifestations of this disease. Dietary factors may influence these processes directly or via a range of cardiovascular disease risk factors. Obesity, particularly when centrally distributed, is associated with an appreciable increase in the risk of coronary heart disease. There is also evidence implicating specific nutrients and, in particular, high intakes of some saturated fatty acids appear to be important promoters of coronary heart disease. On the other hand, there is increasing evidence of a strong protective effect by a range of antioxidant nutrients. Increasing carbohydrate intake can assist in the reduction of saturated fat and many fruits and vegetables rich in carbohydrates are also rich in several antioxidants. Cereal foods rich in non-starch polysaccharides have been shown to be protective against coronary heart disease in a series of prospective studies. There is no evidence for a causal role of sucrose in the etiology of coronary heart disease. The cornerstone of dietary advice aimed at reducing coronary heart disease risk is to increase the intake of carbohydrate-rich foods, especially cereals, vegetables and fruits rich in non-starch polysaccharide, at the expense of fat. Among those who are overweight or obese it is more important to reduce total fat intake and to encourage the consumption of the most appropriate carbohydrate-containing foods. There has been concern that a substantial increase in carbohydrate-containing food at the expense of fat, might result in a decrease in high-density lipoprotein and an increase in very low-density lipoprotein and triglycerides in the blood. There is, however, no evidence that this occurs when the increase in carbohydrates results from increased consumption of vegetables, fruits and appropriately processed cereals, over prolonged periods.

Certain non-starch polysaccharides (for example β-glucans) have been shown to have an appreciable effect in lowering serum cholesterol when consumed in naturally occurring foods, or foods which have been enriched by purified forms, or even when fed as dietary supplements. Such polysaccharides may be used in the management of patients with existing hypercholesterolemia but their role, if any, in the prevention of coronary heart disease remains to be established.

Less information is available concerning the role of carbohydrates in other cardiovascular diseases. Plant foods are good sources of potassium and reducing the sodium to potassium ratio may help to reduce the risk of hypertension. Limited data suggest a protective effect of vegetables and fruit in cerebrovascular disease.

There has been considerable debate in many developed countries which have high rates of coronary heart disease regarding the age at which children should start to reduce fat intake towards the recommended level for adults. Clearly children require an adequate intake of energy for growth, and it is important that this does not include an excessive intake of carbohydrates at a very young age. It is generally accepted that dietary carbohydrate should gradually be increased and fat reduced after the age of two years, so that by the age of five years children should have reached a diet in the range of that recommended for adults. This advice should, of course, include the key dietary guidelines for children and adolescents, which suggest that nutritional adequacy should be achieved by eating a wide variety of foods and that energy intake should be adequate to promote growth and development, and to reach and maintain desirable body weight.

Cancer

Diet is widely regarded as important in the etiology of colorectal cancer with meat and fat considered the primary risk factors, and fruit, vegetable and cereal foods considered to be protective. Cancer is a disease associated with well-recognized genetic abnormalities and for colorectal cancer in particular, defects in a number of genes have been clearly defined (67,80). These genes mostly code for proteins responsible for the control of either cell growth, cell-to-cell communication or DNA repair. They are mainly oncogenes or tumour suppressor genes. For the development of colorectal cancer an individual must acquire several of these genetic abnormalities in the same cell. The acquisition of gene defects in somatic cells is thought to be through DNA damage and a resultant failure of the DNA repair system (or of apoptosis). Dietary carbohydrate is thought to be protective through mechanisms involving arrest of cell growth, differentiation and selection of damaged cells for cell death (apoptosis). This is probably achieved primarily through the action of butyric acid which is formed in the colon from fermentation of carbohydrates such as resistant starch and non-starch polysaccharides. Such carbohydrates are found mostly in cereals, fruit and vegetables.

The process of fermentation may protect the colorectal area against the genetic damage that leads to colorectal cancer through other mechanisms which include: a) the dilution of potential carcinogens; b) the reduction of products of protein fermentation through stimulation of bacterial growth; c) pH effects; d) maintenance of the gut mucosal barrier; and, e) effects on bile acid degradation. These mechanisms, however, are much less well-established.

Carbohydrate staple foods are a source of phytoestrogens which may be protective for breast cancer. Cancer risk is increased for the obese. This applies especially to cancers of the breast and uterus. However, this is a general effect of total energy intake and not specifically of carbohydrates. Dietary carbohydrates do not have a known role in the etiology of lung, breast, stomach, prostate, pancreas, oesophagus, liver or cervical cancers. There is, however, some evidence that there is an increased risk of ovarian cancer in women with mild galactosemia (81,82).

Gastrointestinal diseases other than cancer

Intakes of non-starch polysaccharides and resistant starch are the most important contributors to stool weight. Therefore, increasing consumption of foods rich in these carbohydrates is a very effective means of preventing and treating constipation, as well as haemorrhoids and anal fissures. Bran and other cereal sources containing non-starch polysaccharide also appear to protect against diverticular disease and have an important role in the treatment of this condition. Obesity is an important risk factor for gallstones. High intakes of carbohydrate may facilitate the colonization of bifidobacteria and lactobacilli in the gut and thus reduce the risk of acute infective gastrointestinal illnesses.

Dental caries

The incidence of dental caries is influenced by a number of factors. Foods containing sugars or starch may be easily broken down by α-amylase and bacteria in the mouth and can produce acid which increases the risk of caries. Starches with a high glycemic index produce more pronounced changes in plaque pH than low glycemic index starch, especially when combined with sugars (20). However, the impact of these carbohydrates on caries is dependent on the type of food, frequency of consumption, degree of oral hygiene performed, availability of fluoride, salivary function, and genetic factors. Prevention programmes to control and eliminate dental caries should focus on fluoridation and adequate oral hygiene, and not on sucrose intake alone.

Other conditions

There are a number of inherited conditions having significant implications for restricted dietary carbohydrate intake in infants and children. These include rare conditions such as galactosemia, fructose intolerance, a wide range of glycogen storage diseases, sucrase deficiencies and monosaccharide transport deficiencies. Though rare in incidence, their early detection and careful dietary management is important if severe handicap or pathology is to be avoided.

CHAPTER 4

THE ROLE OF THE GLYCEMIC INDEX IN FOOD CHOICE

Carbohydrate foods often contain vitamins and minerals plus other compounds, such as phytochemicals and antioxidants, which may have health implications. Consuming a wide variety of carbohydrate foods is therefore recommended as this is more likely to be a nutritionally adequate diet with the health benefits commonly ascribed to carbohydrate foods (83).

Food choice depends not only on nutrition and health considerations but also on factors such as local availability, cultural acceptability and individual likes and needs. There is no one measure which can be used to guide food choices in all cases. The chemical composition of foods (e.g. fat, sugars, dietary fibre content) should be an important factor influencing food choice. However, simply knowing the chemical nature of the carbohydrates in foods, for example, does not reliably indicate their actual physiologic effects. Foods which are good choices in some situations may not be the best choices in others. Likewise, foods which are poor choices in some situations may be good choices in others.

Two indices of carbohydrate foods based on their physiologic functions have been proposed. A recently suggested satiety index (84) measures the satiety value of equal energy portions of foods relative to a standard, which is white bread. The factors which control food intake are complex and satiety needs to be distinguished from satiation. Nevertheless, investigation of satiety indices of foods is considered an interesting area of future research, which, if validated, may aid in the selection of appropriate carbohydrate foods to promote energy balance. A more established index is the glycemic index which can be used to classify foods based on their blood glucose raising potential.

Definition of glycemic index (GI)

The glycemic index is defined as the *incremental area* under the *blood glucose* response curve of a *50g carbohydrate portion* of a test food expressed as a percent of the response to the same amount of carbohydrate from a *standard food* taken by the *same subject*. The italicized terms are discussed below because the methods used to determine the glycemic index of foods and to apply the information to diets may profoundly affect the results obtained.

Incremental area under the curve

A number of different methods have been used to calculate the area under the curve. For most glycemic index data, the area under the curve has been calculated as the incremental area under the blood glucose response curve (IAUC), ignoring the area beneath the fasting concentration. This can be calculated geometrically by applying the trapezoid rule. When a blood glucose value falls below the baseline, only the area above the fasting level is included. Sample data are shown in Table 1. The data for Standard #1 are used in the diagram in Figure 2 to illustrate the details of the actual calculation.

TABLE 1
Sample blood glucose responses to the ingestion of 50g carbohydrate

Minutes	0	15	30	45	60	90	120	IAUC
Standard #1	4.3	6.3	7.9	5.3	4.1	4.6	4.9	114
Standard #2	4.0	6.0	6.7	5.5	5.3	5.0	4.2	155
Standard #3	4.1	5.8	8.0	6.5	5.9	4.8	3.9	179
Test Food	4.0	5.0	5.8	5.4	4.8	4.2	4.4	93

50g carbohydrate portion:

The portion of food tested should contain 50g of glycemic (available) carbohydrate. In practice, glycemic carbohydrate is often measured as total carbohydrate minus dietary fibre, as determined by the AOAC method. Since this method does not include RS1 and RS2 when they are present, they will be mistakenly included as glycemic carbohydrate.

Blood glucose response

This is normally measured in capillary whole blood. Plasma glucose can be used to determine the glycemic index and gives similar values. However, capillary blood is preferred because it is easier to obtain, the rise in blood glucose is greater than in venous plasma and the results for capillary blood glucose are less variable than those for venous plasma glucose. Thus, differences between foods are larger and easier to detect statistically using capillary blood glucose (85). An illustration of the difference between glucose as measured in simultaneously-obtained venous plasma and capillary whole blood is shown in Table 2.

TABLE 2
Glucose response from capillary blood and venous plasma

	0min	15min	30min	45min	60min	90min	120min	IAUC
Capillary blood	4.1	6.3	9.0	8.7	6.7	5.7	3.9	279
Venous plasma	5.0	7.1	8.8	8.0	5.6	5.4	4.2	155

Standard food

Either white bread or glucose can be used as the standard food. The GI values obtained if white bread is used are about 1.4 times those obtained if glucose is the standard food. Other standard foods could be used, but to enable comparison with data in the literature, the GI of the new standard food relative to standardized white bread or glucose should be established.

Same subject

Blood glucose responses vary considerably from day-to-day within subjects. Thus, to obtain a representative mean response to the standard food, it is recommended that the standard food be repeated at least three times in each subject. This is illustrated by the data in Table 1, which is typical for normal subjects. The standard food was repeated three times giving IAUCs of: 114, 155 and 179. The mean±SD IAUC is 149±33 and the coefficient of variation (100×SD/mean) is 22%. For this subject, the GI of the test food = 100×93/149 = 62.

Figure 2

Sample calculations of incremental area under the curve (IAUC)

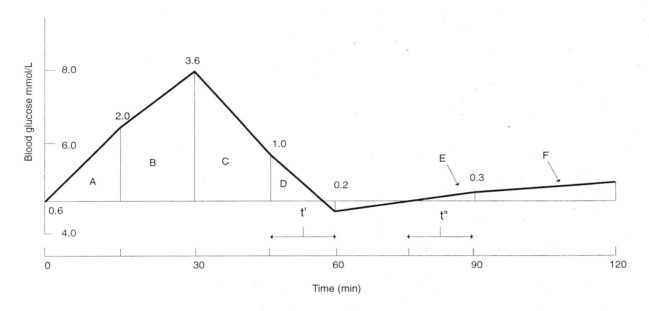

The IAUC for the data illustrated above (Standard #1, Table 3) equals the sum of the areas of the triangles and trapezoids: A+B+C+D+F

The area of triangle A = 2.0 x 15/2 = 15.0
The area of trapezoid B = (2.0 + 3.6) x 15/2 = 42.0
The area of trapezoid C = (3.6 + 1.0) x 15/2 = 34.5
The area of triangle D = 1.0 x t'/2
   since: t'/15 = 1.0/(1.0 + 0.2)
   therefore: t' = 15 x 1.0/1.2 = 12.5
   therefore the area of triangle D = 1.0 x 12.5/2 = 6.25
The area of triangle E = 0.3 x t"/2
   since: t"/30 = 0.3/(0.3 + 0.2)
   therefore: t" = 30 x 0.3/0.5 = 18
   therefore the area of triangle D = 0.3 x 18/2 = 2.7
The area of trapezoid F = (0.3 + 0.6) x 30/2 = 13.5

Therefore, IAUC = 15.0 + 42.0 + 34.5 + 6.25 + 2.7 +13.5 = 114 mmol.min/L

Protocol

To determine the GI of the food, the tests illustrated in Table 1 would be repeated in six or more subjects and the resulting GI values averaged. Normally, the GI for more than one food would be determined in one series of tests, for example, each subject might test four foods once each and the standard food three times for a total of seven tests in random order on separate days. Subjects are studied on separate days in the morning after a 10-12 hour overnight fast. A standard drink of water, tea or coffee should be given with each test meal.

Factors influencing the blood glucose responses of foods

Starchy foods with a low GI are digested and absorbed more slowly than foods with a high GI. Some factors that influence glycemic properties of foods are listed in Table 3.

TABLE 3
Food factors influencing glycemic responses

Amount of carbohydrate

Nature of the monosaccharide components
> Glucose
> Fructose
> Galactose

Nature of the starch
> Amylose
> Amylopectin
> Starch-nutrient interaction
> Resistant starch

Cooking/food processing
> Degree of starch gelatinization
> Particle size
> Food form
> Cellular structure

Other food components
> Fat and protein
> Dietary fibre
> Antinutrients
> Organic acids

Calculation of glycemic index of meals or diets

The GI can be applied in a detailed fashion to mixed meals or whole diets by calculating the weighted GI value of the meal or diet. For example, the way to calculate the GI of a meal containing bread, cereal, sucrose, milk and orange juice is shown in Table 4.

TABLE 4
Calculation of the glycemic index of meals

Food	Grams Glycemic Carbohydrate	Proportion of total Glycemic Carbohydrate	Food Glycemic Index	Meal Glycemic Index*
Bread	25	0.342	100	34.2
Cereal	25	0.342	72	24.6
Milk	6	0.082	39	3.2
Sucrose	5	0.068	87	5.9
Orange juice	12	0.164	74	12.1
TOTAL	73			80.0

* Values for each food equals the proportion of total glycemic carbohydrate multiplied by the food GI. The sum of these values is the meal GI.

Using this type of calculation, there is a good correlation between meal GI and the observed glycemic responses of meals of equal nutrient composition. Blood glucose responses are also influenced by the amount of carbohydrate in the meal. To compare the expected glycemic load of meals with different carbohydrate contents, a non-linear adjustment can be applied (86), but this has only been tested in normal subjects.

For detailed application of the GI, a value of the GI for every food in the diet or meal needs to have been assigned (for many foods the value has to be estimated). The accuracy of the calculation depends upon the accuracy of the GI values ascribed to foods, which may vary from place to place due to local factors such as variety, cooking, processing, etc. Foods particularly prone to such variation include rice, potatoes and bananas.

Practical application of the glycemic index

The glycemic index can be used, in conjunction with information about food composition, to guide food choices. For practical application, the glycemic index is useful to rank foods by developing exchange lists of categories of low glycemic index foods, such as legumes, pearled barley, lightly refined grains (e.g. whole grain pumpernickel bread, or breads made from coarse flour), pasta, etc. Specific local foods should be included in such lists where information is available (e.g. green bananas in the Caribbean and specific rice varieties in Southeast Asia).

In choosing carbohydrate foods, both glycemic index and food composition must be considered. Some low GI foods may not always be a good choice because they are high in fat. Conversely, some high GI foods may be a good choice because of convenience or because they have low energy and high nutrient content. It is not necessary or desirable to exclude or avoid all high GI foods.

Physiologic and therapeutic effects of low glycemic index foods

Meals containing low GI foods reduce both postprandial blood glucose and insulin responses. Animal studies suggest that incorporating slowly digested starch into the diet delays the onset of insulin resistance. Some epidemiologic studies suggest that a low GI diet is associated with reduced risk of developing non-insulin diabetes in men (87) and women (88). Clinical trials in normal, diabetic and hyperlipidemic subjects show that low GI diets reduce mean blood glucose concentrations, reduce insulin secretion and reduce serum triglycerides in individuals with hypertriglyceridemia (89,90,91,92). In addition, the digestibility of the carbohydrate in low GI foods is generally less than that of high GI foods. Thus, low GI foods increase the amount of carbohydrate entering the colon and increase colonic fermentation and short chain fatty acid production. This has implications for systemic nitrogen and lipid metabolism, and for local events within the colon.

CHAPTER 5

GOALS AND GUIDELINES FOR CARBOHYDRATE FOOD CHOICES

Rationale and framework

Although the scientific basis for dietary guidelines requires an understanding of physiology and health relationships, the guidance most helpful to consumers uses food-based terms (93). In preparing such guidelines, food traditions and beliefs must be taken into account and the total food intake should reflect practical issues, such as meal patterns, food status, celebratory or usual role, seasonal availability, affordability and sustainability. These, including the health priorities, are matters for national policy makers.

Principles of carbohydrate food choices

The principles are:

1. To acknowledge the socio-cultural context, lifestyle and stage of life-cycle, in food carbohydrate choice;

2. To give preference to food choices rather than to nutrient goals in carbohydrate food choices, and in so doing:

   a. Use food categories as a guide to chemically defined carbohydrate type.

   b. Use numbers of portions (serving sizes) of foods from designated food categories in order to provide semi-quantitative food-based advice. This may imply that meal frequency would need to increase in some cultures, because the accommodation of enough carbohydrate food in the course of the day, without an excessive amount on any one occasion, requires more frequent servings and consumption;

3. To appreciate that many of the world's health problems are associated with inadequate carbohydrate intake, and potentially also associated with inappropriate carbohydrate intake;

4. To ensure the acceptability and practicality of any recommended change in carbohydrate food intake;

5. To acknowledge that there may be unintended consequences involved in carbohydrate food intake change, and also to ensure that risks involved in dietary changes from traditional diets is considered;

6. To monitor the intake of carbohydrate foods and, wherever possible, of chemically defined carbohydrate components of those foods in relation to health issues.

7. To ascertain whether food carbohydrate choices encourage biodiversity and are sustainable.

Carbohydrate nutrient and food goals

Nutrient goals

The minimum amount of carbohydrate in the human diet that is needed to avoid ketosis is of the order of 50 g/day in adults. Beyond this, additional energy needs are best met by nutrient-dense carbohydrate foods. There must, of course, be adequate intakes of protein (with essential amino acids) and essential fatty acids from fat. Moderate intake of sugar-rich foods can also provide for a palatable and nutritious diet.

Food goals

There are a number of approaches to translating nutrient recommendations to food goals:

1. Recommending the total weight of food groups to be consumed. Various national food guides have suggested quantities of specific foods to be consumed, such as fruits and vegetables, and pulses, nuts and seeds.

2. Examining sources of carbohydrate foods in various diets, particularly diets which have desirable total carbohydrate intakes or from countries where the incidence of lifestyle diseases is low. Recommendations can then be made on the basis of intakes.

3. Examining major food groups which contain carbohydrate foods and recommending numbers of servings of those food groups. Numerous countries around the world, both developed and developing, have produced food guides with such groupings, and considering the level of agreement that exists for carbohydrate as a percent energy, these food guides are remarkably consistent in their advice.

4. Examining indices which exist to describe various physiological properties of carbohydrate-containing foods, such as glycemic index values and values from other indices which are presently being developed.

On the basis of the above approaches, and taking into account the principles for carbohydrate food choice, the following recommendations can be made:

1. A variety of foods should provide the carbohydrate in the diet, not a single or small number of sources.

2. Cereals, roots, pulses, fruit and vegetables are all components of a healthy diet throughout the world.

3. Cereal foods or root crops, where this is the main staple, should provide the major source of carbohydrate energy.

4. Intake of fruits and vegetables (including potatoes in developed countries) should be high. As well as being a valuable source of carbohydrate, fruit and vegetables are an important source of antioxidant vitamins and other food components.

5. Consumption of pulses, nuts and seeds should be encouraged. While this group often represents only a small amount of carbohydrate energy, these foods are a good source of protein and micronutrients. They should be consumed with cereals to optimize protein quality.

6. At least small quantities of milk products are desirable, even when low lactase activity exists, since these are a good source of protein and micronutrients.

These recommendations apply to all individuals over the age of two years, with adjustments as necessary for growth and the increased demand of pregnancy and lactation.

Translation from carbohydrate nutrients to foods

Achieving goals for intake of carbohydrates does not ensure nutritional adequacy. Carbohydrate foods provide a range of nutrients and other substances essential for health in addition to energy. It is therefore essential to consume a variety of foods in order to derive the full benefits of a high carbohydrate diet. Nutrients from foods require monitoring. For example, in Iran (94) carbohydrate foods include vegetables (250 g/day), fruits (210 g/day), pulses (20 g/day) and cereals (wheat at about 250 g/day and rice 110 g/day, uncooked). Wheat has mostly been consumed as bread with traditional pastries being festive foods. Recently, consumption of the latter has increased substantially with potential reduction of nutritionally useful food groups traditionally accompanying bread. This may not significantly impact on total carbohydrate intake, but could influence nutritional adequacy. Traditional methods of food preparation and preservation facilitate food choice variety, and promote nutritional benefits. Alteration of traditional practices may compromise such benefits. Ongoing monitoring may be required to guard against nutritional inadequacy.

Considerations for target audiences

Planners and policy makers need to:

1. Recognize dietary goals of at least 55% of total energy from a variety of carbohydrate sources.

2. Recognize the extent of change necessary in order to meet these goals (e.g. it may take considerable change in food production and consumption to meet goals in Western countries).

3. Understand that there must be a gradual transition in meeting new dietary guidelines and that new terminology will need to be gradually accepted.

4. Consider the effects of economic and cultural factors in achieving dietary goals.

5. Develop clear guides about the types and quantities of food recommended.

6. Develop methods to monitor food consumption to meet dietary goals.

Primary producers and processors need to:

1. Consider how existing and new technologies can be used to help meet dietary goals regarding the quantity and nutritional properties of food carbohydrates, as well as levels of micronutrients and other desirable food components.

2. Provide foods, such as breakfast cereals and snack foods that are high in NSP, low in energy density, and with a low glycemic index.

3. Increase the availability and convenience of fruits and vegetables.

4. Provide appropriate information to the consumer on food labels.

To facilitate individual choice

Provide easily understandable food-based guides for the consumer.

CHAPTER 6
RECOMMENDATIONS

The following recommendations are derived from the Consultation discussions and resulting conclusions detailed in the report. Specific recommendations are grouped under the appropriate report headings.

The role of carbohydrates in nutrition

The Consultation RECOMMENDS:

1. That the terminology used to describe dietary carbohydrate be standardized with carbohydrates classified primarily by molecular size (degree of polymerization or DP) into sugars (DP 1-2), oligosaccharides (DP 3-9) and polysaccharides (DP 10+). Further subdivision can be made on the basis of monosaccharide composition. Nutritional groupings can then be made on the basis of physiological properties.

2. That the concept of glycemic carbohydrate, meaning "providing carbohydrate for metabolism" be adopted.

3. Against the use of the terms extrinsic and intrinsic sugars, complex carbohydrate and available and unavailable carbohydrate.

4. That food laboratories measure total carbohydrate in the diet as the sum of the individual carbohydrates and not "by difference".

5. That the use of the term dietary fibre should always be qualified by a statement itemizing those carbohydrates and other substances intended for inclusion. Dietary fibre is a nutritional concept, not an exact description of a component of the diet.

6. That the use of the terms soluble and insoluble dietary fibre be gradually phased out. The Consultation recognized that these terms are presently used but does not consider them a useful division either analytically or physiologically

7. That the analysis and labelling of dietary carbohydrate, for whatever purpose, be based on the chemical divisions recommended. Additional groupings such as polyols, resistant starch, non-digestible oligosaccharides and dietary fibre can be used, provided the included components are clearly defined.

8. That the energy value of all carbohydrate in the diet be reassessed using modern nutritional and other techniques. However, for carbohydrates which reach the colon, the Consultation recommends that the energy value be set at 2 kcal/g (8 kJ/g) for nutritional and labelling purposes.

9. That the continued production and consumption of root crops and pulses be encouraged to ensure the adequacy and diversity of the supply of carbohydrate.

10. That the continued consumption of traditional foods rich in carbohydrate should be encouraged where populations are in transition from a subsistence rural economy to more prosperous urban lifestyles. Processed foods are likely to be a substantial part of the diet and processing can be used to optimize nutritional properties.

The role of carbohydrates in the maintenance of health

The Consultation RECOMMENDS:

11. That the many health benefits of dietary carbohydrates should be recognized and promoted. Carbohydrate foods provide more than energy alone.

12. An optimum diet of at least 55% of total energy from a variety of carbohydrate sources for all ages except for children under the age of two. Fat should not be specifically restricted below the age of 2 years. The optimum diet should be gradually introduced beginning at 2 years of age.

13. That energy balance be maintained by consuming a diet containing at least 55% total energy from carbohydrate from various sources and engaging in regular physical activity.

14. Against consuming carbohydrate levels above the optimum, including carbohydrate-containing beverages, for purposes of recreational physical activity. Higher carbohydrate intakes are only needed for long-term extreme endurance physical activities.

15. That, as a general rule, a nutrient-dense, high carbohydrate diet be considered optimal for the elderly, but that individualization is recommended because their specific nutritional needs are complex.

Dietary carbohydrate and disease

The Consultation RECOMMENDS:

16. That a wide range of carbohydrate-containing foods be consumed so that the diet is sufficient in essential nutrients as well as total energy, especially when carbohydrate intake is high.

17. That the bulk of carbohydrate-containing foods consumed be those rich in non-starch polysaccharides and with a low glycemic index. Appropriately processed cereals, vegetables, legumes, and fruits are particularly good food choices.

18. That excess energy intake in any form will cause body fat accumulation, so that excess consumption of low fat foods, while not as obesity-producing as excess consumption of high fat products, will lead to obesity if energy expenditure is not increased. Excessive intakes of sugars which compromise micronutrient density should be avoided. There is no evidence of a direct involvement of sucrose, other sugars and starch in the etiology of lifestyle-related diseases.

19. That national governments provide populations in transition from traditional diets to those characteristic of developed countries, with dietary recommendations to ensure nutritional adequacy and retention of an appropriate balance of macronutrients.

The role of glycemic index in food choice

The Consultation RECOMMENDS:

20. That for healthy food choices, both the chemical composition and physiologic effects of food carbohydrates be considered, because the chemical nature of the carbohydrates in foods does not completely describe their physiological effects.

21. That, in making food choices, the glycemic index be used as a useful indicator of the impact of foods on the integrated response of blood glucose. Clinical application includes diabetes and impaired glucose tolerance. It is recommended that the glycemic index be used to compare foods of similar composition within food groups.

22. That published glycemic response data be supplemented where possible with tests of local foods as normally prepared, because of the important effects that food variety and cooking can have on glycemic responses.

REFERENCES

1. FAO. 1980. Carbohydrates in human nutrition, a Joint FAO/WHO Report. *FAO Food and Nutrition Paper 15*, Rome.

2. Asp, N-G. 1996. Dietary carbohydrates: classification by chemistry and physiology. *Food Chemistry* 57:9-14.

3. Cummings, J.H., Roberfroid, M.B., Andersson, H., Barth, C., Ferro-Luzzi, A. 1997. A new look at dietary carbohydrate: chemistry, physiology and health. *European Journal of Clinical Nutrition*, 52:1-7.

4. Englyst, H.N. and Hudson, G.J. 1996. The classification and measurement of dietary carbohydrates. *Food Chemistry*, 57(1):15-21.

5. Southgate, D.A.T. 1991. *Determination of food carbohydrates.* Elsevier Science Publishers, Ltd, Barking.

6. Greenfield, H. and Southgate D.A.T. 1992. *Food composition data. Production, management and use.* Elsevier Applied Science, London.

7. Asp, N.-G. 1995. Classification and methodology of food carbohydrates as related to nutritional effects. *American Journal of Clinical Nutrition* 61(4(S)):930S -937S.

8. Department of Health. 1989. *Dietary sugars and human health.* Her Majesty's Stationery Office, London.

9. U.S. Senate Select Committee on Nutrition and Human Needs. 1977. *Dietary goals for the United States.* 2nd Ed. U.S. Government Printing Office, Washington D.C.

10. McCance, R.A. and Lawrence, R.D. 1929. The carbohydrate content of foods. *Medical Research Council Special Report Series* 135 Her Majesty's Stationery Office, London.

11. Englyst, H.N. and Cummings, J.H. 1990. Non-starch polysaccharides (dietary fiber) and resistant starch. *New Developments in Dietary Fiber. Physiological, Physicochemical, and Analytical Aspects.* (Furda, I. and Brine, C.J. eds.). Plenum Press, New York and London, pp. 205-225.

12. Englyst, H.N., Kingman, S.M. and Cummings, J.H. 1992. Classification and measurement of nutritionally important starch fractions. *European Journal of Clinical Nutrition* 46:S33-S50.

13. Wurzburg, O.B. 1986. Nutritional aspects and safety of modified food starches. *Nutrition Reviews* 44:74-79.

14. Björck, I., Gunnarsson, A. and Östergård, K. 1989. *A study of native and chemically modified potato starch. Part II. Digestibility in the rat intestinal tract.* Stärke 41:128-134.

15. Trowell, H. 1972. Dietary fibre and coronary heart disease. *Revue Européenne d'Etudes Cliniques et Biologiques* 17(4) 345-349.

16. Burkitt, D.P. and Trowell, H.S. 1975. *Refined carbohydrate foods and disease: some implications of dietary fibre.* Academic Press, London.

17. British Nutrition Foundation. 1990. *Complex carbohydrates in foods: report of the British Nutrition Foundation's Task Force.* Chapman and Hall, London.

18. Asp, N-G., Schweizer, T.F., Southgate, D.A.T. and Theander, O. 1992. Dietary fibre analysis. In *Dietary fibre. A component of food. Nutritional function in health and disease* (eds. T.F. Schweizer and C.A. Edwards), Springer, London, pp. 57-102.

19. Muir, J. and O'Dea, K. 1993. Validation of an in vitro assay for predicting the amount of starch that escapes digestion in the small intestine of humans. *American Journal of Clinical Nutrition* 57:546.

20. Björck, I. 1996. Starch: nutritional aspects, In: *Carbohydrates in food* (Eliasson A-C. ed.), Marcel Dekker Inc, pp 505-554.

21. Asp, N-G., van Amelsvoort, J.M.M. and Hautvast, J.G.A.J. 1996. (eds.) Nutritional implications of resistant starch. *Nutrition Research Reviews* 9, 1-31 (final EURESTA report).

22. Englyst, H.N., Quigley, M.E. Hudson, G.J. and Cummings, J.H. 1992. Determination of dietary fibre as non-starch polysaccharides by gas-liquid chromatography. *Analyst*, 117:1707-1714.

23. Englyst, H.N., Quigley, M.E. and Hudson, G.J. 1994. Determination of dietary fibre as non-starch polysaccharides with gas-liquid chromatographic, high-performance liquid chromatographic or spectrophotometric measurement of constituent sugars. *Analyst*, 119:1497-1509

24. Pendlington, A.W. and Brookes, A. 1995. BCR studies in progress. In: Recent progress in the analysis of dietary fibre. COST 92 *Metabolic and physiological aspects of dietary fibre in food.* European Commission. Directorate-General XII Science, Research and Development, Luxemburg, ISBN 92-827-4981-9, p.p. 129-141.

25. Englyst, H.N., Quigley, M.E., Englyst, K.N., Bravo, L. and Hudson, G.J. 1996. Dietary fibre. Measurement by the Englyst NSP procedure. Measurement by the AOAC procedure. Explanation of the differences. *J. Assoc. Publ. Analysts*, 32:1-52.

26. *FAOSTAT* (PC version) [CD-ROM]. 1996. Available: Food and Agriculture Organisation, Rome.

27. Grigg, D. International variations in food consumption in the 1980's. *Geography* 1993;78:251-66.

28. Grigg, D. The starchy staples in world food consumption. *Annals of the Association of American Geographers* 1996; 86:412-431.

29. Cho, W.J. Changing food consumption and dietary intake in AFO countries. *Report of an APO Symposium*, December 1994. Asia Productivity Organization, 1996.

30. Scrimshaw, N.S., Taylor, L. Food. *Scientific American* 1980;243:78-88.

31. Stoskopf, N.C. *Cereal grain crops.* Reston, VA: Reston Publishing Co., Inc., 1985.

32. Dyson, T. *Population and Food.* London: Routledge, 1996.

33. Food and Agriculture Organization. In: *World agriculture: Towards 2010, an FAO study* (ed. N. Alexandratos), London: J. Wiley & Sons, 1995.

34. Dowler, E.A., Ok Seo, Y.I. Assessment of energy intake. *Food Policy* 1985; August:278-88.

35. Gibson, R.S. *Principles of nutritional assessment.* New York: Oxford University Press, 1990.

36. Crane, N.T., Lewis, C.J., Yetley, E.A. Do time trends in food supply levels of macronutrients reflect survey estimates of macronutrient intake? *American Journal of Public Health* 1992;82:862-6.

37. Stephen, A.M., Wald, N.J. Trends in individual consumption of dietary fat in the United States, 1920-1984. *American Journal of Clinical Nutrition*; 52:457-69.

38. Stephen, A.M., Sieber, G.M. Trends in individual fat consumption in the United Kingdom 1900-1988. *British Journal of Nutrition* 1994;71:775-788.

39. Stephen, A.M., Sieber, G.M., Gerster, Y.A., Morgan, D.R. Intake of carbohydrate and its components - international comparisons, trends over time and effects of changing to low fat diets. *American Journal of Clinical Nutrition* 1995;62:851S-67S.

40. Gregory, J., Foster, K., Tyler, H., Wiseman, M. *The dietary and nutritional survey of British adults.* London: HMSO, 1990.

41. Commonwealth Department of Community Services and Health. *National dietary survey of adults: 1983. No. 2 Nutrient intakes.* Canberra: Australian Government Publishing Service, 1987.

42. Commonwealth Department of Community Services and Health. *National dietary survey of schoolchildren (aged 10-15 years): 1985. No. 2 Nutrient intakes.* Canberra:Australian Government Publishing Service, 1989.

43. Morgan, K.J., Zabik, M.E. Amount and food sources of total sugar intake by children ages 5 to 12 years. *American Journal of Clinical Nutrition* 1981;34:404-13.

44. Gibson, S.A. Consumption and sources of sugars in the diets of British schoolchildren: Are high-sugar diets nutritionally inferior? *Journal of Human Nutrition and Dietetics* 1993;6:355-71.

45. Englyst, H.N., Cummings, J.H. Improved method for measurement of dietary fibre as non-starch polysaccharides in plant foods. *Journal of the Association of Official Analytical Chemists* 1988;71:808-14.

46. Cummings, J.H., Frolich, W. eds. *Dietary fibre intakes in Europe.* Brussels: Commission of the European Community, 1993.

47. Kuratsune, M., Honda, T., Englyst, H.N., Cummings, J.H. Dietary fiber in the Japanese diet as investigated in connection with colon cancer risk. *Japanese Journal of Cancer Research.* 1986;77:736-8.

48. Amaral, M.L.K. *Dietary fibre and lipid metabolism.* PhD Thesis, University of Saskatchewan, Canada. 1995.

49. Prosky, L., Asp, N-G., Furda, I., DeVries, J.W., Schweizer, T., Harland, B. Determination of total dietary fiber in foods, food products and total diets: Interlaboratory study. *Journal of the Association of Official Analytical Chemists* 1984;67:1044-52.57.

50. Southgate, D.A.T. Determination of carbohydrates in foods. II. Unavailable carbohydrate. *Journal of the Science of Food and Agriculture* 1969;20:331-5.

51. Bursztyn, P.G. A diet survey in Zimbabwe. *Human Nutrition. Applied Nutrition* 1985; 39A:376-88.

52. Campbell, T.C., Junshi, C. Diet and chronic degenerative diseases: perspectives from China. *American Journal of Clinical Nutrition* 1994;59:1153S-61S.

53. Beegom, R., Beegom, R., Niaz, M.A., Singh, R.B. Diet, central obesity and prevalence of hypertension in the urban population of South India. *International Journal of Cardiology* 1995;51:183-91.

54. Livesey, G. and Elia, M. 1995. *Short chain fatty acids as an energy source in the colon: metabolism and clinical implications. Physiological and clinical aspects of short chain fatty acids*, (J.H. Cummings, J.L. Rombeau and T. Sakata, eds.) Cambridge University Press, Cambridge, 472-482.

55. Roberfroid, M., Gibson, G.R. and Delzenne, N. 1993. The biochemistry of oligofructose, a non-digestible fibre: an approach to calculate its caloric value. *Nutrition Reviews*, 51:137-146.

56. Blundell, J.E., Green, Sue and Burley, Victoria. 1994. Carbohydrates and human appetite. *American Journal of Clinical Nutrition* 59:728S-734S.

57. Rolls, B.J. and Hammer, V.A. 1995. Fat, carbohydrate and the regulation of energy intake. *American Journal of Clinical Nutrition* 62:1086S-1095S.

58. Levin, R.J. 1994. Digestion and absorption of carbohydrates - from molecules and membranes to humans. *American Journal of Clinical Nutrition.* 59: 690S-698S.

59. Buller, H.A. and Grand, R.J. 1990. Lactose intolerance. *Annual Review of Medicine*, 41:141-148.

60. Gudmand-Hoyer, E. 1994. The clinical significance of disaccharide maldigestion. *American Journal of Clinical Nutrition.* 59:735S-741S.

61. Dills, W.L. 1993. Protein fructosylation: fructose and the Maillard reaction. *American Journal of Clinical Nutrition* 58(5(S)):779S-787S.

62. MacDonald, R.B. 1995. Influence of dietary sucrose on biological aging. *American Journal of Clinical Nutrition* 62(1(S)):284S-293S.

63. Lairon, D. 1994. *Mechanisms of action of dietary fibre on lipid and cholesterol metabolism.* Commission of the European Communities, Luxembourg.

64. Truswell, A.S. 1994. Food carbohydrates and plasma lipids - an update. *American Journal of Clinical Nutrition* 59(3(S)):710S-718S.

65. Heijnen, M-L.A., Van Amelsvoort, J.M.M., Deurenberg, P. and Beynen, A.C. 1996. Neither raw nor retrograded starch lowers fasting serum cholesterol levels in healthy, normolipidemic subjects. *American Journal of Clinical Nutrition* 64:312-318.

66. Cummings, J.H. and Macfarlane, G.T. 1991. The control and consequences of bacterial fermentation in the human colon. *Journal of Applied Bacteriology,* 70:443-459.

67. Cummings, J.H. 1997. The large intestine in nutrition and disease. *Danone Chair Monograph* 103-110, Institute Danone, Bruxelles.

68. Cummings, J.H. and Macfarlane, G.T. 1997. The role of intestinal bacteria in nutrient metabolism. *Clinical Nutrition*, 16:3-11.

69. Gibson, G.R. and Roberfroid, M. 1995. Dietary modulation of the human colonic microbiota: introducing the concept of prebiotics. *Journal of Nutrition,* 125:1401-1412.

70. Thomas, C.D., Peters, J.C., Reed, G.W., Abumrad, N.N., Sun, M., and Hill, J.O. 1992. Nutrient balance and energy expenditure during ad libitum feeding of high-fat and high-carbohydrate diets in humans. *American Journal of Clinical Nutrition* 55:934-942.

71. Stubbs, R.J., Harbron, C.G., Murgatroyd, P.R. and Prentice, A.M. 1995. Covert manipulation of dietary fat and energy density: Effect on substrate flux and food intake in men eating ad libitum. *American Journal of Clinical Nutrition* 62:316-329.

72. Flatt, J.P. 1993. Dietary fat, carbohydrate balance and weight maintenance. *Annals of the New York Academy of Sciences* 683:122-140.

73. Horton, T.J., Drougas, H., Brachey, A., Reed, G.W., Peters, J.C. and Hill, J.O. 1995. Fat and carbohydrate overfeeding in humans: Different effects on energy storage. *American Journal of Clinical Nutrition* 62:19-29.

74. Schwarz, J.M., Neese, R.A., Turner, S., Dare, D. and Hellerstein, M.K. 1995. Short-term alterations in carbohydrate energy intake in humans - Striking effects on hepatic glucose production, de novo lipogenesis, lipolysis and whole-body fuel selection. *Journal of Clinical Investigation* 96:2735-2743.

75. Bergstrom, J. and Hultman, E. 1966. Muscle glycogen synthesis after exercise: an enhancing factor localized to the muscle cells in man. *Nature* 210:309.

76. Vaisman, N., Voet, H., Akivis, A. and Vakil, E. 1996. Effect of breakfast timing on the cognitive functions of elementary school students. *Archives of Pediatrics and Adolescent Medicine* 150:1089-1092.

77. White, J.W. and Wolraich, M. 1995. Effect of sugar on behavior and mental performance. *American Journal of Clinical Nutrition* 62:S242-S249.

78. FAO/WHO. 1994. Codex Alimentarius, Volume 4, Foods for special dietary uses. *STAN 72-1981, Codex Standard for Infant Formula.* FAO, Rome.

79. Zimmet, P., Dowse, G., Finch, C. *et al.* 1990. The epidemiology and natural history of NIDDM; lessons from the South Pacific. *Diabetes/Metabolism Reviews* 6:91-124.

80. Cummings, J.H. 1994. Nutritional management of diseases of the stomach and bowel. *Human Nutrition and Dietetics*, (J.S. Garrow and W.P.T. James, eds.) Churchill Livingston, London: 480-506.

81. Cramer, D.W., Muto, M.G., Reichardt, J.K., Xu, H., Welch, W.R., Valles, B. and Ng, W.G. 1994. Characteristics of women with a family history of ovarian cancer. I. Galactose consumption and metabolism. *Cancer* 74(4):1309-1317.

82. Kaufman, F.R., Devgan, S., and Donnell, G.N. 1993. Results of a survey of carrier women for the galactosemia gene. *Fertility and Sterility* 60(4):727-728.

83. Hodgson, J.M., Hsu-Hage, B.H. and Wahlqvist, M.L. 1994. Food variety as a quantitative descriptor of food intake. *Ecology of Food and Nutrition*, 32:137-148.

84. Holt, S.H.A., Brand Miller, J.C. and Petocz, P. 1996. Interrelationships among postprandial satiety, glucose and insulin responses and changes in subsequent food intake. *Euopean Journal of Clinical Nutrition*, 50:788-797.

85. Wolever, T.M.S. and Bolognesi, C. 1996. Source and amount of carbohydrate affect postprandial glucose and insulin in normal subjects. *Journal of Nutrition* 126:2798-2806.

86. Wolever, T.M.S. and Bolognesi, C. 1996. Prediction of glucose and insulin responses of normal subjects after consuming mixed meals varying in energy, protein, fat, carbohydrate and glycemic index. *Journal of Nutrition* 126:2807-2812.

87. Salmerón, J., Ascherio, A., Rimm, E.B., Colditz, G.A., Spiegelman, D., Jenkins, D.J., Stampfer, M.J., Wing, A.L. and Willet, W.C. 1997. Dietary fiber, glycemic load and risk of NIDDM in men. *Diabetes Care*, 20:545-550.

88. Salmerón, J., Stampfer, M.J., Colditz, G.A., Manson, J.E., Wing, A.L. and Willet, W.C. 1997. Dietary fiber, glycemic load and risk of non-insulin-dependent diabetes mellitus in women. *Journal of the American Medical Association*, 277:472-477.

89. Wolever, T.M.S., Jenkins, D.J.A., Jenkins, A.L. and Josse, R.G. 1991. The glycemic index: methodology and clinical implications. *American Journal of Clinical Nutrition* 54:846-854.

90. Wolever, T.M.S. 1997. The glycemic index: Flogging a dead horse? *Diabetes Care* 20:452-456.

91. Wolever, T.M.S., Jenkins, D.J.A., Vuksan, V., Jenkins, A.L., Buckley, G.C., Wong, G.S. and Josse, R.G. 1992. Beneficial effect of a low-glycemic index diet in type 2 diabetes. *Diabetic Medicine* 9:451-458.

92. Frost, G., Keogh, B., Smith, D., Akinsanya, K. and Leeds, A. 1996. The effect of low-glycemic carbohydrate on insulin and glucose response in vivo and in vitro in patients with coronary artery disease. *Metabolism* 45:669-672.

93. FAO/WHO. 1996. Preparation and use of food-based dietary guidelines. *Report of a Joint FAO/WHO Consultation, Nicosia, Cyprus.* WHO/NUT/96.6. Geneva.

94. Kimiagar, S.M., Ghaffarpour, M., Hormozyari, H., Mohammed, K., Eslam, F. and Noronzi, F. 1995. *Nationwide household food consumption pattern survey report.* Ministry of Health, and Centre for Agriculture Planning and Economic Studies, Ministry of Agriculture. Tehran.

Annex 1

Intake of Carbohydrate and Its Components

Intake of Carbohydrate and Its Components, Individual Countries by Continent Since 1980

Country	Year	n	Energy kcal	Carbohydrate g	Carbohydrate % energy	Starch g	Starch % energy	Sugars g	Sugars % energy
Africa - adults									
Malawi (1)	1997	141	1457	287	78.7	-	-	-	-
Nigeria (2)	1987	67	2540	324	51.0	-	-	-	-
South Africa -black (3)	(1995)	61	1969	278	57.2	-	-	-	-
South Africa- black (4)	1990	649	1665	228	55.7	-	-	-	-
So. Africa - coloured (5)	1990	976	1981	224	45.2	147	29.7	77	15.6
Zimbabwe -white (6)	1985	99	2226	217	39.0	113	20.3	53*	9.5*
Zim. - black urban (6)	1985	91	2345	287	49.0	186	31.7	62*	10.6*
Zim. - black rural (6)	1985	49	2590	351	54.2	260	40.2	60*	9.2*
Africa -children									
South Africa (7)	1982	843	2058	262	50.9	-	-	-	-
Asia - adults									
Bangladesh (8)	1981-82	3141	1943	431	88.7	-	-	-	-
China (9)	1982	103,662	2963	514	69.4	-	-	-	-
China (10)	1983-84	6500	2650	473	71.4	-	-	-	-
China (11)	1992	3682	2396	355	59.3	-	-	-	-
India (12)	1983-84	563	2093	301	57.5	-	-	-	-
Philippines (13)	1985	400	1767	300	67.9	-	-	-	-
Vietnam (14)	1988	7462	1998	407	81.5	-	-	-	-
Asia - children									
China (10)	1982	63,343	-	368	-	-	-	-	-
Europe - adults									
Belgium (15)	1980-85	10,971	2473	240	38.9	144	23.3	97	15.7
France (16)	1988	25	1969	209	42.5	-	-	-	-
Hungary (17)	1990-92	2559	2799	314	44.9	207	29.6	107	15.3
Netherlands (18)	1987-88	4134	2309	244	42.2	122	21.1	119	20.6
Netherlands (19)	(1990)	107	2221	228	41.1	116	20.9	112	20.2
UK (20)	1986-87	2197	2061	232	42.3	130	25.2	100	19.4
Europe - children									
Netherlands (18)	1987-88	1409	2256	271	48.0	121	21.5	148	26.2
UK (21)	1980	405	2050	261	50.9	144	28.1	117	22.8
UK (22)	1981	120	2190	280	51.1	158	28.9	122	22.3
UK (23)	1986-87	4760	2369	278	46.9	154	26.0	124	20.9
UK (21)	1990	379	2015	258	51.2	139	27.6	119	23.6
Latin America - adults									
Chile (36)	1995	859	1981	287	58.0	-	-	-	-
North America - adults									
Canada (24)	1989	96	2053	269	52.2	-	-	-	-
Canada (25)	1989	2212	2070	244	47.1	-	-	-	-
Canada (37)	1990	2118	2196	262	47.7	-	-	-	-
USA (26)	(1984)	155	2570	240	37.4	105	16.3	35*	5.5*
USA (27)	1976-80	11864	1882	254	54.0	-	-	-	-
USA (27)	1988-91	7931	2109	244	46.3	-	-	-	-
North America - children									
USA (28)	1988	1463	1613	202	50.1	104	25.8	99	24.6
USA (27)	1976-80	8102	1830	227	49.6	-	-	-	-
USA (27)	1988-91	5999	1806	238	52.7	-	-	-	-
Oceania - adults									
Australia (29)	1983	6255	2190	232	42.4	125	22.8	107	19.5
New Zealand (30)	1992	-	2105	233	44.3	-	-	101	19.2
Papua New Guinea (31)	1991	750	2628	406	61.8	349	53.1	57	8.7
Solomon Islands (32)	1985	1071	2508	442	70.5	-	-	-	-
Oceania - children									
Australia (33)	1985	5224	2049	259	50.6	129	25.2	130	25.4
Australia (34)	1986	141	1666	208	49.9	99	23.8	108	25.9
New Zealand (35)	1993	251	1946	263	54.0	130	26.7	133	27.3

* sucrose only

Note: Most countries in Africa, Asia, and North America calculate carbohydrate 'by difference'. Most countries in Europe and Oceania analyse carbohydrate directly. Values for Europe and Oceania therefore do not contain unavailable carbohydrate, while values for Africa, Asia and North America do. Method of deriving carbohydrate is rarely given

References cited in the foregoing table

1. Gibson R.S. 1997. Personal communication.

2. Adams-Campbell L.L., Agurs, T.D. and Ukoli, F.A. 1993. Dietary assessment in Nigerian women: a pilot study. *Ethnicity and Disease.* 3:S62-S66.

3. Vorster H.H., Venter, C.S., Menssink, E., van Staden, D.A., Labadarios, D., Strydom, A.J.C., Silvis, N., Gericke, G.J. and Walker, A.R.P. 1994. Adequate nutritional status despite restricted dietary variety in adult rural vendas. *South African Journal of Clinical Nutrition* 7:3-16.

4. Bourne, L.T., Langenhoven, M.L., Steyn, K., Jooste, P.L., Laubscher, J.A. and Van der Vyver, E. 1993. Nutrient intake in the African population of the Cape Peninsula, South Africa: the BRISK study. *Central Africa Journal of Medicine* 39:238-247.

5. Steyn, K., Langenhoven, M.L., Joubert, G., Chalton, D.O., Benade, A.J.S. and Rossouw, J.E. 1990. The relationship between dietary factors and serum cholesterol values in the coloured population of the Cape peninsula. *South African Medical Journal* 78:63-67.

6. Bursztyn, P.G. 1985. A diet survey in Zimbabwe. *Human Nutrition. Applied Nutrition* 39A:376-388.

7. Steyn, N.P., Albertse, E.C., Van Wyck Kotze, T.J. and Van Heerden, L., 1986. Analysis of the diets of 12-year old children in Cape Town. *South African Medical Journal.* 69:739-742.

8. FAO. 1987. ESN - *Nutrition country profile - Bangladesh.* Food and Agriculture Organization, Rome.

9. FAO. 1989. ESN - *Nutrition country profile - China.* Food and Agriculture Organization, Rome.

10. Campbell, T.C. and Junshi, C., 1994. Diet and chronic degenerative diseases: perspectives from China. *American Journal of Clinical Nutrition.* 59:1153S-1161S.

11. Tian, H.G., Nan, Y., Hu, G., Dong, X.L., Pietinen, Y.P. and Nissinen, A. 1995. Dietary survey in a Chinese population. *European Journal of Clinical Nutrition* 49:26-32.

12. Beegom, R., Niaz, M.A. and Singh, R.B. 1995. Diet, central obesity and prevalence of hypertension in the urban population of South India. *International Journal of Cardiology.* 51:183-191.

13. FAO. 1988. ESN - *Nutrition country profile - Philippines.* Food and Agriculture Organization, Rome.

14. FAO. 1994. ESN - *Apercu nutritionnel - Vietnam.* Food and Agriculture Organization, Rome.

15. Kornitzer, M. and Bara, L. 1989. Clinical and anthropometric data, blood chemistry and nutritional patterns in the Belgian population. *Acta Cardiologica* 44:101-144.

16. Asciutti-Moura, L.S., Guilland, J.C., Fuchs, F., Richard, D. and Klepping, J. 1988. Fatty acid composition of serum lipids and its relation to diet in an elderly institutionalised population. *American Journal of Clinical Nutrition* 48:980-987.

17. Biro, G., Antal, M. and Zajkas, G. 1996. Nutrition survey of the Hungarian population in a randomised trial between 1992-1994. *European Journal of Clinical Nutrition* 50:201-208.

18. Löwik, M.R.H., Brussaard, J.H., Hulshof, K.F.A.M., Kistemaker, C., Schaafsma, G., Ockhuizen, T. and Hermus, R.J.J., 1994. Adequacy of the diet in the Netherlands in 1987-88 (Dutch nutrition surveillance system). *International Journal of Food Sciences and Nutrition*. 45:S1-S62.

19. Goldbohm, R.A., vanden Brandt, P.A., Brants, H.A.M., van't Veer, P., Al, M., Sturmans, F. and Hermus, R.J.J. 1994. Validation of a dietary questionnaire used in a large-scale prospective cohort study on diet and cancer. *European Journal Clinical Nutrition* 48:253-265.

20. Gregory, J., Foster, K., Tyler, H. and Wiseman, M. 1990. *The dietary and nutritional survey of British adults*. Her Majesty's Stationery Office, London.

21. Adamson, A., Rugg-Gunn, A., Butler, T., Appleton, D. and Hackett, A. 1992. Nutritional intake, height and weight of 11-12 year old Northumbrian children in 1990 compared with information obtained in 1980. *British Journal of Nutrition*. 68:543-563.

22. Rugg-Gunn, A.J., Hackett, A.F., Jenkins, G.N. and Appleton, D.R. 1991. Empty calories? Nutrient intake in relation to sugar intake in English adolescents. *Journal of Human Nutrition and Dietetics* 4:101-111.

23. Lorenz, K.J. and Kulp, K. 1991. *Handbook of cereal science and technology*. Marcel Dekker, Inc., New York.

24. Amaral, M.L.K. 1993. *Dietary fibre and lipid metabolism*. PhD Thesis, University of Saskatchewan, Canada. Nova Scotia Heart Health Program. Nova Scotia Nutrition Survey. Nova Scotia Department of Health, Halifax, Canada.

25. Nova Scotia Heart Health Program. 1993. *Nova Scotia heart health survey*. Nova Scotia Department of Health, Halifax, Canada.

26. Dreon, D.M., Frey-Hewitt, B., Ellsworth, N., Williams, P.T., Terry, R.B. and Wood, P.D. 1988. Dietary fat:carbohydrate ratio and obesity in middle-aged men. *American Journal of Clinical Nutrition* 47:995-1000.

27. Life Sciences Research Office, FASEB. 1995. *Third report on nutrition monitoring in the United States*. US Government Printing Office, Washington D.C.

28. Nicklas, T.A., Webber, L.S., Koshak, M. and Nerenson, G.S. 1992. Nutrient adequacy of low fat intakes for children: the Bogalusa heart study. *Pediatrics* 89:221-228.

29. Commonwealth Department of Community Services and Health. 1987. *National dietary survey of adults: 1983. No. 2 Nutrient intakes*. Australian Government Publishing Service, Canberra.

30. Wilson, N.C., Allen, J.B., Russell, D.G. and Herbison, P. 1993. Nutrient analysis II of 24 hour diet recall using 1992 DSIR database. *Report No. 93-26. Life in New Zealand* activity and Health Research Unit, University of Otago, Dunedin, New Zealand.

31. Hodge, A.H., Dowse, G.K., Koki, G., Mavo, B., Alpers, M.P. and Zimmet, P.Z. 1995. Modernity and obesity in coastal and highland Papua New Guinea. *International Journal of Obesity* 19:154-161.

32. Eason, R.J., Pada, J., Wallace, R., Henry, A. and Thornton, R. 1987. Changing patterns of hypertension , diabetes, obesity and diet among Melanesians and Micronesians in the Solomon Islands. *Medical Journal of Australia.* 146:465-473.

33. Commonwealth Department of Community Services and Health. 1989. *National dietary survey of schoolchildren (aged 10-15 years): 1985. No. 2 Nutrient intakes.* Australian Government Publishing Service, Canberra.

34. Magarey, A.A., Nicholas, J. and Boulton, J. 1987. Food intake at age 8. 1. Energy, macro- and micronutrients. *Australian Paediatric Journal* 23:173-178.

35. George, J., Brinsdon, S.C., Paulin, J.M. and Aitken, E.F. 1993. What do young adolescent New Zealanders eat? Nutrient intakes of nationwide sample of Form 1 children. *New Zealand Medical Journal* 106:47-51.

36. Castillo, C., Atalah, E., Benavides, X. and Urteaga, C. 1997. Patrones alimentarios en adultos que asisten a consultorios de la Region Metropolitana. *Revista Medica de Chile* 125:283-289.

37. Santé Québec. 1995. Les Québécoises et les Québécois mangent-ils mieux*? Rapport de l'enquête québécoise sur la nutrition.* Gouvernement du Québec, Montréal.

Annex 2

Background Information

INTRODUCTION

The following background information has been developed from the background papers prepared for the Consultation. Extracts have been taken from those papers and they have been edited, condensed, and in some cases combined in order to provide contextual information for the decisions and recommendations of the Consultation.

Each section provides an overview of specific areas of discussion as well as information and data that should prove useful to workers in the field. In their original form, the papers were too voluminous for inclusion in this publication. The information they provided was reduced in size through judicious editing in an attempt to keep the text simple and factual.

The literature citations for each paper have been grouped together in numerical sequence in a references section at the end of this Annex.

GLOBAL TRENDS IN PRODUCTION AND CONSUMPTION OF CARBOHYDRATE FOODS

Introduction

The term "carbohydrate" describes a family of contributing compounds, all constructed from the same monosaccharide building blocks, ranging from the simple sugars, or mono and disaccharides, through sugar alcohols, oligosaccharides and dextrins, to the more complex starch and non-starch polysaccharides. With this wide array of compounds, it follows that there are a considerable number of food sources which contribute to the total carbohydrate in the diet.

Trends in food production, availability and consumption

A number of approaches can be used to examine trends in both supply and intake of foods and nutrients, these are:

1. Production

2. Food balance sheets

3. Household surveys

4. Individual assessments

For worldwide comparisons and trends over time, any of the above approaches can be used, and each has both advantages and limitations.

Production

Production is extremely useful in examining trends throughout the world. Production figures are available from FAO for every country in the world for every crop (1). Most countries produce food for their own consumption, and in addition are net food importers. Only a small number of countries are major exporters of carbohydrate foods, primarily grains. These include the United States, Canada, Argentina, Australia, Thailand and Viet Nam.

Crop yield is affected by agricultural practices, weather conditions and external forces. Agricultural practices, such as improved crop varieties, increased land use, increased irrigation of land, or increased use of fertilizers, herbicides, and insecticides can all result in increased yield, and all have contributed to the increases in crop production over the last three decades (see Figure 1).

No matter how good the cultivar or the growth conditions, however, environmental conditions can have an overriding effect on yield. Generally, drought, excess water, cold, hail, and wind account for about 90% of all crop losses (2), with drought by far the major factor. This can clearly be seen with production of cereals in North America in the late 1980's, particularly 1988, when continued lack of rain and minimal snow cover in wheat-growing areas of the United States and Canada had a severe effect on crop production.

External forces, in the form of the organizational structure of the country and its political stability are all factors affecting agricultural production. Wars and political unrest have a major effect on agriculture and can result in marked reductions in crop production. This has been seen in many countries when unrest occurs.

Figure 1

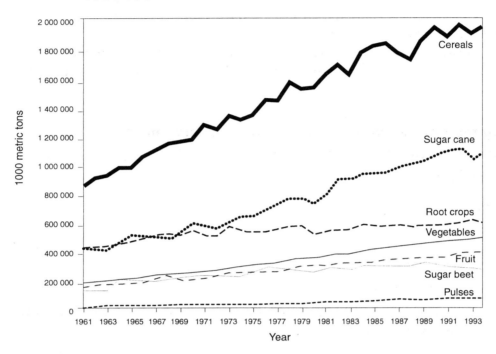

Major sources of carbohydrate - world production 1961-1994

Food Balance Sheets

Food balance sheets are available for every country in the world, for every food item (1). These are converted to nutrients based on the composition of the individual food commodities included in the production data. Food balance is typically calculated by taking into account the quantity of foodstuffs produced in a country, added to the quantity imported and adjusted for any changes in stocks that have occurred. In order to determine the food available for human consumption, all other food uses must be taken into account. These include the quantity of food exported, fed to livestock, used for seed, and used for non-food use. Even food losses during storage and transportation must be considered.

Food balance sheets, although describing consumption of foods or nutrients per capita of the population for a country, do not represent food actually consumed. They cannot determine waste at a variety of levels, including the home. Food balance sheets in prosperous or developed countries are therefore an overestimate of food actually consumed, while in many developing countries, with little food waste, they are closer to actual consumption or even less than consumption because of home production (3).

Household surveys

Household surveys and individual data, therefore, represent the closest to food actually consumed. With increasing food consumption outside the home, however, household data, such as the continuing National Food Survey in the UK, has recently become much less meaningful and reflective of food actually consumed than in past decades. Like food balance, household surveys may also not be able to evaluate wastage and spoilage, although efforts have been made to take account of wastage in the home (4).

Individual assessments

Individual surveys represent the best way to assess food actually consumed. However, they also have limitations. First, they are not available for all countries. Many countries, particularly in the developing world, do not have the resources to mount large nutrition surveys, or even small studies on specific groups.

In the developed world, many countries do conduct national surveys, and these provide an invaluable source of data for food and nutrient intake. Some countries, like the United States, conduct national surveys on a regular basis as a government requirement, but most do so only sporadically because of the large cost involved. In spite of their infrequent nature, national surveys are the major source of reliable information on actual dietary intake around the world. These are supplemented by small surveys in single locations on smaller numbers of individuals. Methodologies vary from one survey to the next, as well as from country to country. In North America, for example, 24 hour recall is the most common method of dietary assessment and is that used most often whereas the UK has used 7 day weighted assessments. These different methods have differing problems, but a problem with both is some degree of underreporting, both intentional and involuntary (4).

In light of the limitations of the various methods for assessing consumption, emphasis has been placed on production and individual assessment data. Although these also have limitations, they are lesser in magnitude and easier to interpret than the errors in food balance and household surveys. Errors in food balance can also vary more with increasing prosperity, than do production and individual assessments and hence comparisons between the developing and developed countries are more difficult when using food balance data.

Carbohydrate foods

The major carbohydrate-containing foods in the human diet are:

     1. Cereals

     2. Sweeteners

     3. Root crops

     4. Pulses

     5. Vegetables

     6. Fruit

     7. Milk products

Cereals

Cereals refer to the graminaceous family, and are considered to be crops harvested for dry grain only. Crops grown for grazing or harvested green for forage or silage are defined as fodder crops. Of the 17 primary cereals defined by FAO, those which make a significant contribution to the human diet are rice, wheat, maize (corn), barley, rye, oats, millet and sorghum. The composition of the major cereals is shown in Table 1. In general, cereals contain 65-75% of their total weight as carbohydrate, 6-12% as protein, and 1-5% fat. Compared to other carbohydrate sources, they are therefore the most nutrient dense. The majority of the carbohydrate is present as starch but cereals are also a major provider of non-starch polysaccharides to the diet and also contain some simple sugars.

TABLE 1
Nutritive value of major cereals /100g edible portion (5-7)

Cereal	Energy kJ	Moisture %	Protein g	Fat g	CHO* g	NSP* g	TDF* g	Starch g	Sugars g
Wheat	1318	14.0	12.7	2.2	63.9	9.0	12.6	61.8	2.1
Maize	1515	12.0	8.7	0.8	77.7	na	11.0	71	1.6
Rice	1531	11.8	6.4	0.8	80.1	2.0	3.5	80.1	1.0
Barley	1282	11.7	10.6	2.1	64.0	14.8	17.3	62.2	1.8
Sorghum	1610	14.0	8.3	3.9	57.4	na	13.8	(50)	1.3
Millet	1481	13.3	5.8	1.7	75.4	na	8.5	60	4
Rye	1428	15.0	8.2	2.0	75.9	11.7	14.6	75.9	na
Oats	1698	8.9	12.4	8.7	72.8	6.8	10.3	72.8	1.2

* CHO = carbohydrate; NSP = Non-starch polysaccharides; TDF = Total dietary fibre

Of the major cereals, maize, wheat and rice are well ahead of the others in terms of production as each of these three grains contributes over 25% to the world's production of cereals. This contribution to total cereals has remained relatively steady over the last thirty years (1). Although maize emerged as the largest crop in 1994, this was the first year it had done so. In developed countries a large proportion of maize is used as feed for livestock, particularly poultry, pigs, and ruminants (8).

Since the 1960's, rice has been produced in the developing world, with over 90% of total world production in these countries, primarily for local consumption (1). Sorghum, too, is a crop of the developing countries with only 30% produced in the developed world. Wheat was traditionally a crop of the developed world, but has undergone considerable change in the last three decades, so that world production is now virtually split between the developing and developed world (1).

Sugar crops

Sugars are the second largest contributor to carbohydrate in the diet throughout the world. The major sources of sugars are sugar cane and sugar beet. Sugars are also produced from other crops where they are derived from starch. This includes high fructose corn syrup (HFCS) made from corn in the US and sugars produced from potatoes in Japan (9,10). Honey, molasses, maple and others are only minor sugar sources. Sugar cane is the predominant source of sucrose, with a production of over 1.3 million metric tons per year, and being a tropical crop, most of this is in the developing countries. Production of sugar cane continues to increase at a rate of some 2% per year. This is largely due to increased yields, rather than increased crop area (9).

Sugar beet is a temperate crop, and production in some parts of the world, particularly Europe, has declined in recent years with the closure of a large number of sugar factories (10). Nevertheless, many European countries are self-sufficient in sugar and import no cane sugar (10). In other countries, most notably the United States, a reduction in use of sucrose from sugar beet and sugar cane has occurred because of increased use of high fructose corn syrup, which in turn resulted from the high price of sucrose for food manufacturing during the 1980s.

Both sugar cane and sugar beet are 10-20% sucrose, generally around 15-16% (10). Hence although sugar cane is the second largest carbohydrate crop (see Figure 1), when it is compared to cereals which are 60-70% carbohydrate, the contribution of sugar cane to total dietary carbohydrate intake is small (about 10-12% of all carbohydrate produced worldwide).

Root Crops

Root crops, or as often described, roots and tubers, are the third largest carbohydrate food sources, although well behind cereals and sugar cane in total tons produced (see Figure 1). The major contributors to root crops are potatoes, cassava (manioc), yams, sweet potatoes and taro. Minor crops such as jicama, chayote and yambeam are consumed in specific countries. The composition of the major root crops is shown in Table 2. Generally root crops contain 15-30% carbohydrate, 1-2% protein and less than 0.5% fat. Like cereals, the majority of carbohydrate in root crops is starch (70-75% dry weight), but they are also excellent sources of non-starch polysaccharide and contain simple sugars (1-3% dry weight) (12,13). With storage, some of the starch in root crops, like cassava, is converted to sugars, so that after 6 weeks, sugars comprise 12-13% dry weight, rather than 1-3% when first harvested (12,13).

TABLE 2
Nutritive value of root crops /100g edible portion (11)

Root crop	Energy kJ	Moisture %	Protein g	Fat g	CHO* g	NSP* g	TDF* g	Starch g	Sugars g
Potato	318	79.0	2.1	0.2	17.2	1.3	1.8	16.6	0.6
Cassava	607	64.5	0.6	0.2	36.8	1.7	na	35.3	1.5
Sweet Potato (yellow)	372	73.7	1.2	0.3	21.3	2.4	3.0	15.6	5.7
Yam	488	67.2	3.0	0.3	28.2	1.3	3.3	27.5	0.7
Taro	451	68.3	1.4	0.2	26.2	2.4	2.9	25.1	1.1

* CHO = carbohydrate; NSP = Non-starch polysaccharides; TDF = Total dietary fibre

World production of the major root crops indicates that potatoes are by far the most important component. Although the proportion of total root crops has been falling in the last 30 years, potatoes still represent nearly half all such crops consumed (1). Potatoes are consumed in large amounts in North America, Eastern and Western Europe, Latin America, and in some countries in Asia, like South Korea, and Turkey (14).

Pulses, vegetables, fruit, other sources

Pulses, vegetables, fruit, and crops grown mainly for oil (such as groundnuts and soybeans), represent other crops which provide carbohydrate for the diet.   In quantitative terms, vegetables and fruit have much greater production figures than pulses, but their carbohydrate content is considerably less, except for bananas and plantains (vegetables: 5-8% carbohydrate, fruit: 8-15%) (15,16). Production of pulses is only a fraction of cereals and root crops, but pulses are very high in carbohydrate (50-60% on a dry weight basis), and are a major contributor to carbohydrate intake in some countries. The composition of those crops having a high carbohydrate content are shown in Table 3.

TABLE 3

Nutritive value of selected pulses, nuts, bananas and plantains /100g edible portion (11,17,18)

Root crop	Energy kJ	Moisture %	Protein g	Fat g	CHO* g	NSP* g	TDF* g	Starch g	Sugars g
Banana	403	75.1	1.2	0.3	23.2	1.1	1.6	2.3	20.9
Plantain	476	68.2	0.9	0.2	29.3	na	na	na	na
Dry peas	1288	13.3	21.6	2.4	52.0	4.7	na	47.6	2.4
Dry bean[†]	1218	11.3	21.4	1.6	49.7	17.0	40.0	42.7	2.8
Chickpea (Garbanzo bean)	1355	10.0	21.3	5.4	49.6	10.7	na	43.8	2.6
Dry broad bean	1041	11.0	26.1	2.1	32.5	6.1	19.0	24.4	5.9
Lentils (green)	1264	10.8	24.3	1.9	48.8	8.9	na	44.5	1.2
Lentils (red)	1353	11.1	23.8	1.3	56.3	4.9	na	50.8	2.4
Soybean	1551	8.5	35.9	18.6	15.8	15.7	na	4.8	5.5
Groundnut (Peanut)	2341	6.3	25.6	46.1	12.5	6.2	8.0	6.3	6.2

*CHO = carbohydrate;   NSP = Non-starch polysaccharides;   TDF = Total dietary fibre
[†] Dry bean, haricot, common bean, kidney bean, navy bean, snap bean, pinto bean - analysed as haricot bean.

Starchy staples

Cereals and root crops constitute the 'starchy staples' in the human diet and as such are the primary source of dietary carbohydrate throughout the world. The contribution of these crops to the diet varies from continent to continent, and even among countries within continents. The consumption of starchy staples throughout the world has changed over the last three decades. Figure 2 shows the world picture of crop distribution, with countries highlighted according to the starchy staple providing the highest proportion of energy (1986-88) (19). As can be seen, large parts of the world depend on wheat and rice, with more selected areas dependent on maize, root crops, sorghum and millet.

Figure 2

Starchy staples providing the highest proportion of food energy, 1990-1992

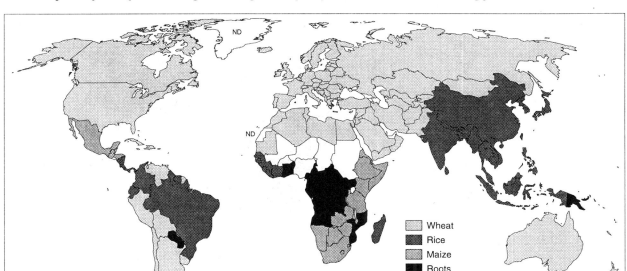

Source: Reproduced with permission from the Geographical Association (19)

The proportion of total energy derived from these same starchy staples around the world are shown in Figure 3 (20). Asia and Africa stand out, with 70% or more of total calories from these major crops. It can clearly be seen why there is a need for production on a large scale in these developing parts of the world.

Food Balance Sheets

Food balance information is of limited usefulness in examining real trends in consumption of foods and nutrients because of changes with growing prosperity. Food balance data for carbohydrates may show little change, for example, while individual assessments over the same time show changing carbohydrate intakes, which mirror changes in fat intake (21,22). One author has indicated that as income increases, consumption of products rich in starch decreases. In developed regions, a rapid fall in the consumption of cereal products, especially bread, is clear as income increases (23).

Developed countries, such as the US and UK, have a much lower per capita carbohydrate consumption than countries in Asia, Africa, and South America. While there may be small shifts in these latter countries, carbohydrate does not appear to be declining to the levels consumed in the developed world. It is important to determine from individual assessments if this is truly the case or if the unmeasurables in food balance data are masking the real picture.

Figure 3

Energy from the dominant starch staples, 1990-1992

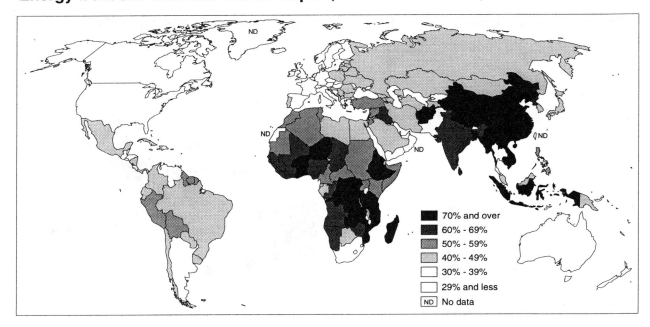

Source: Reproduced with permission from the Association of American Geographers (20)

While food balance data may be subject to considerable error in terms of absolute consumption, it can give a reasonable picture of the distribution of sources contributing to the overall intake of a nutrient. This is shown for carbohydrate in Table 4, for the developing and developed countries, and for the entire world. It can be clearly seen that cereals make the greatest contribution to carbohydrate intake throughout the world, with sweeteners in second place followed by other carbohydrate foods. Overall the total energy provided by carbohydrate to the diet is similar throughout the world; however, the percent energy represented by carbohydrate is considerably lower in the developed countries, because of higher intakes of protein and fat.

Individual Assessments

Individual assessments would seem to provide the most accurate way of determining intake of foods and nutrients. As already mentioned, however, this data is not available on a regular basis for most countries, and for some, hardly at all. In addition to this irregular availability, much of the difficulty in comparing carbohydrate intake around the world is that in many countries carbohydrate is calculated in foods "by difference". Carbohydrate values determined this way are obtained by subtracting the weight of the other major components in a food, namely moisture, fat, protein, and ash, from the total weight of a food. What remains is said to be carbohydrate.   There are several problems with this method.   Firstly, it does not represent direct analysis of carbohydrate, and means that any errors in the estimation of the other nutrients will result in an error in the carbohydrate value. Secondly, there is no description of the individual carbohydrates and with growing interest in various types of carbohydrate (for example, sugars, oligosaccharides or starch), the limitation of a single carbohydrate figure is obvious. Thirdly, "carbohydrate by difference" figures include "unavailable carbohydrate" (dietary fibre) which has a different energy value and different physiological properties than the digestible components of carbohydrate.

TABLE 4
Energy from carbohydrate by food group and as a % of total carbohydrate.
Food balance data - 1964 and 1994

	Developed countries				Developing countries				World			
	......1964.......		......1994.......		......1964.......		......1994.......		......1964.......		......1994.......	
	kcal/ cap/d*	% CHO *	kcal/ cap/d	% CHO	kcal/ cap/d	% CHO	kcal/ cap/d	% CHO	kcal/ cap/d	% CHO	kcal/ cap/d	% CHO
Cereals	1053	59.0	866	54.2	1069	71.3	1284	73.3	1029	66.2	1189	69.2
Root Crop	156	8.7	121	7.6	157	10.5	128	7.3	156	10.0	126	7.3
Sweetener	369	20.7	397	24.8	124	8.3	183	10.5	200	12.9	232	13.5
Pulses	26	1.5	17	1.1	72	4.8	48	2.7	58	3.7	41	2.4
Vegetable	40	2.2	47	2.9	22	1.5	30	1.7	28	1.8	34	2.0
Fruit	71	4.0	85	5.3	42	2.8	58	3.3	52	3.3	65	3.8
Milk	70	3.9	65	4.1	14	0.9	20	1.1	32	2.1	30	1.7
Total CHO	**1785**	**100**	**1598**		**1500**	**100**	**1751**	**100**	**1555**	**100**	**1717**	**100**
Total food	**3040**		**3206**		**2030**		**2573**		**2344**		**2718**	
% CHO	58.7		49.8		73.8		68.1		66.3		63.2	

* kcal/cap/d = kilocalories per person per day; CHO = Carbohydrate

Increasing evidence suggests that the diets of Western countries should be more like those in the developing countries, and many countries have recommended that carbohydrate should represent at least 50-55% energy (24-27). The question arises - has carbohydrate intake always been lower in developed countries than developing, or has this occurred only relatively recently? Examination of individual assessments from countries where numerous individual assessments are conducted can help answer this question. The clearest picture is seen for the UK. Detailed dietary assessments have been conducted in the UK since the turn of the century. Carbohydrate intake represented over 60% energy in the 1920's, and apart from a plateau and even a rise, due to rationing during and after the Second World War, carbohydrate intake continued to decrease in the UK, reaching a low of 45-46% energy in the 1950's, 60's and 70's (21,22). With interest in dietary fibre in the 1970's and more recently a renewed interest in starch, intakes of carbohydrate in the UK in the late 1980's, early 1990's have risen to about 48% energy (21,22). By comparison, carbohydrate data from food balance figures for the UK have been stable at 50-51% energy, and do not show the downward and upward trends which have occurred.

Trends and comparisons of carbohydrate components
In spite of the problems with terminology and differences in usage in different parts of the world, it is possible to collate some studies to gain a picture of what is happening to intake of components of carbohydrate over time, and from country to country. The lack of information

in published work emphasizes the need for researchers to publish dietary information from surveys in more detail, and not simply to publish a paper which contains only nutrients of interest at the time of publication. Those studies which have a lasting impact are those where information has been provided on many nutrients.

Sugars

Sucrose data obtained from Canada and the United States suggest that sucrose intake is declining in North America. As indicated earlier, however, the increased use of high fructose corn syrup as a sweetener is not included in US data for sucrose, and therefore, data on total sugars is what is required to gain a clearer picture of the situation. For the United Kingdom, where sugars are expressed as all free sugars in the diet (as percent energy), the trend has been in an upward direction in recent years. Again, there is a shortage of data for long term trends, but the recent trend is clear and the UK data has the advantage of consistency in measurement, since only one food composition table is used throughout the country.

Clearly more data is needed, since the recent upward trend in the UK in sugars as percent energy, may reflect an increased intake, or it may simply reflect a decreased intake in fat and total energy. Absolute intake in sugars and as a percent energy are identical for the UK and Australia. Australians, however, consume considerably more of their sugars as fruit than in the UK, where sweetened baked goods, sugar itself and sugar products contribute much more to the diet.

Starch

Very few studies report starch intakes, and there are rather too few to consider trends reliably; the upward trend for North America would suggest that intake is heading in a desirable direction. As indicated earlier, however, this may reflect no change in absolute intake, but only an increasing proportion in relation to decreased total energy. Intake of starch is very similar in the UK and Australia, and as would be expected, cereals, particularly breads and breakfast cereals, and potatoes make the major contribution to starch intakes in these western diets. As would be expected, starch intakes are considerably higher in countries dependent on starchy staples to a greater degree, such as China, and Japan. There is a need for more individual studies to solidify starch intake estimates.

Dietary Fibre

Dietary fibre intake data from around the world are difficult to compare because of methodology differences. One author derived non-starch polysaccharides for a number of countries and concluded that these did not vary as much as did intakes of starch (28). In fact, the variations between countries may well be due mainly to method differences, rather than to actual variation in intake. It cannot be stressed enough that uniformity in measurement is required before country comparisons of any nutrient intake is possible.

Some discrepancies in reported dietary fibre intake between different countries may be explained by what is included or not included under "cereals". It is clear that cereals and vegetables are the predominant sources of fibre in the diet, and within these categories, bread and potatoes stand out as major contributors.

Resistant Starch

A new component of interest is resistant starch (RS), which is considered to be that starch which resists digestion and absorption in the small intestine and escapes into the colon (29). There have been recent efforts to assess the amount of RS in diets in Europe and Australia. Some of these have only estimated RS_3 (retrograded amylose), which is one of 3 or 4 components of resistant starch in the diet (29,30). Cereals are the greatest source of resistant starch, at 35% or more (30). Resistant starch intakes were calculated for a number of countries in Europe, with an average intake of 4.2 g/d, ranging from 3.2 g/d for Norway to 5.7 g/d for Spain. Of this, cereals accounted for 42% of the RS and potatoes 27% (30). Estimates from some Asian countries , however, are much higher in total, and represent closer to 5% of all starch eaten (30). More analysis is needed of those countries with high intakes of starchy staples, particularly if these are cooked and cooled as in traditional eating practices.

Conclusion

There is growing interest in carbohydrate and its components throughout the world, and recommendations have been made to encourage increased carbohydrate consumption. Assessment of components of particular interest, whether these be sugars, starch, resistant starch or dietary fibre, are hampered by lack of data. This is mainly because of long-standing approaches to carbohydrate measurement, which are indirect and hence inadequate. The reason that this has not been rectified in recent decades is probably due to a lack of recognition of the importance of individual carbohydrate components to health, a situation that continues to this day in some countries. Where interest has grown, as with dietary fibre, a number of different methodologies have emerged which measure different things and therefore give different answers. Comparison of countries is then almost as difficult as if there were no data at all. Comparison of intakes, trends over time, and projections for the future, require uniform methods and good reporting of data. The health implications for populations of physiological findings on small groups, can only be determined if there is knowledge of present consumption. All efforts should be made to ensure that data is collected and is reported in as comprehensive and consistent a manner as possible.

DIETARY CARBOHYDRATE COMPOSITION

Introduction

While a formal definition of a carbohydrate can be considered somewhat difficult, one commonly accepted by chemists is that carbohydrates are "polyhydroxy aldehydes, ketones, alcohols, acids, their simple derivatives and their polymers having polymeric linkages of the acetal type" (31). Carbohydrates are further classified according to their degree of polymerization (DP) as: sugars (mono- and di-saccharides), oligosaccharides (contain three to nine monosaccharide units), and polysaccharides (contain ten or more monosaccharide units) (32).

Carbohydrates play a major role in human diets, comprising some 40-75% of energy intake. Their most important nutritional property is digestibility in the small intestine. In terms of their physiological or nutritional role, they are often classified as available and unavailable carbohydrates. Available carbohydrates are those that are hydrolyzed by enzymes of the human gastrointestinal system to monosaccharides that are absorbed in the small intestine and enter the pathways of carbohydrate metabolism. Unavailable carbohydrates are not hydrolyzed by endogenous human enzymes, although they may be fermented in the large intestine to varying extents.

The carbohydrates in foods of greatest importance are shown in Table 5 (32,33). Small amounts of other carbohydrates can be detected in some foods but these are of little overall significance. These include maltose, commonly formed from hydrolysis of starch and found in starch hydrolyzates used as food ingredients; galactose from fermented dairy products; and pentoses, such as xylose and arabinose, from fruits.

TABLE 5
The most important carbohydrates in foods

Monosaccharides	Glucose, Fructose
Disaccharides	Sucrose, Lactose
Oligosaccharides	Raffinose, Stachyose, Fructo-oligosaccharides
Polysaccharides	Cellulose, Hemicelluloses, Pectins, β-Glucans, Fructans, Gums, Mucilages, Algal polysaccharides
Sugar alcohols	Sorbitol, Mannitol, Xylitol, Lactitol , Maltitol

Monosaccharides

Glucose (also called dextrose) is found in varying amounts in honey, maple syrup, fruits, berries, and vegetables. Glucose is often formed from the hydrolysis of sucrose, as in honey, maple sugar, and invert sugar. It is also present in foods containing starch hydrolysis products, such as corn syrups and high-fructose corn syrups. The amount of glucose contained in these starch hydrolysates depends on the method used in their preparation, e.g. acid conversion, acid-enzyme conversion, or enzyme conversion (34). Small amounts of glucose are also found in maltodextrins and corn syrup solids, commonly used as ingredients in food products.

The physicochemical properties of glucose that are important in its use as a food ingredient include flavour, sweetness, hygroscopicity, and humectancy (35). It is about 70-80% as sweet as sucrose. Since glucose is a reducing sugar, i.e. contains a carbonyl function at the C-1 position, it readily undergoes the Maillard or browning reaction with amino acids. This behaviour is responsible for the golden-brown colour of bread crusts and for the caramel colour and flavour observed in certain other foods. If the reaction is sufficiently extensive, dark brown colours and altered flavours can result in food products.

Fructose is present in honey, maple sugar, fruits, berries and vegetables. Fructose is often present from the hydrolysis of sucrose, as in honey, maple sugar, and invert sugar. It may also be present in food products, such as soft drinks, bakery products, and candies from the use of invert sugar, crystalline fructose or high-fructose corn syrups (HFCS). HFCS are often used as a sweetening agent, particularly in carbonated soft drinks. Fructose is 140% sweeter than sucrose (35). As a keto-hexose, fructose is very reactive with amino acids in the Maillard or browning reaction.

Disaccharides

Sucrose (α-D-glucopyranosyl β-D-fructofuranoside or β-D-fructofuranosyl α-D-glucopyranoside) is a nonreducing sugar and is the major disaccharide in most diets. It is present in honey, maple sugar, fruits, berries, and vegetables. It may be added to food products as liquid or crystalline sucrose or as invert sugar (if not completely inverted to fructose and glucose). It is commercially prepared from sugar cane or sugar beets. Sucrose can provide a number of desirable functional qualities to food products including sweetness, mouth-feel, and the ability to transform between amorphous and crystalline states (35). Sucrose often cannot be easily replaced by other sweeteners due to its lack of aftertaste, browning, and gummy mouth-feel and its characteristic body, viscosity and sweetness profile. This is particularly true in baked products where equivalent replacement, particularly with high intensity sweeteners, often results in a product with decreased textural characteristics and consumer acceptance. Sucrose and invert sugar are used in many food products including ice cream, baked goods, desserts, confections, intermediate-moisture foods, and soft drinks. Its use in soft drinks has decreased because of the increased usage of high-fructose corn syrups due to availability and lower costs.

Lactose (4-O-β-D-galactopyranosyl-D-glucose), a reducing sugar also known as milk sugar, occurs in milk and milk products. It may also occur in food products that contain dairy products as ingredients, such as doughnuts, wafer cookie bars, breakfast bars, and hamburger buns. Whey is used as an ingredient in foods and is high in lactose content. Lactose crystallizes easily and is often responsible for the grittiness encountered in ice cream when crystallization is not inhibited. Lactose serves as an energy source for infants during the nursing period. Lactose is hydrolyzed in the small intestine by the enzyme lactase to galactose and glucose which are then absorbed.

Oligosaccharides

Oligosaccharides are not widely occurring or of great importance in foods and food products, except for a series of galactosylsucroses (often designated as α-galactosides) and fructo-oligosaccharides. The galactosylsucrose family of oligosaccharides include raffinose (a trisaccharide), stachyose (a tetrasaccharide), and verbascose (a pentasaccharide). In vegetables, such as peas, beans, and lentils, the content of these oligosaccharides can range from five to eight percent on a dry matter basis (36). Raffinose, stachyose, and verbascose are not digested in the small intestine by human gastrointestinal enzymes. They are passed into the large intestine where they are fermented by intestinal microflora with the production of gas. It is this behaviour that produces the flatulence for which the consumption of beans is noted. Enzyme preparations are commercially available which can be taken with meals to reduce the tendency for flatulence production by promoting the hydrolysis of these oligosaccharides to constituent monomers which are absorbed.

Fructo-oligosaccharides occur in wheat, rye, triticale, asparagus, onion, and Jerusalem artichoke and a number of other plants. Fructo-oligosaccharides and higher molecular weight fructans can comprise 60-70% of the dry matter in Jerusalem artichokes. Fructo-oligosaccharides have been commercially prepared by the action of a fructofuranosyl furanosidase from Aspergillus niger on sucrose. They are about 30% as sweet as sucrose, have a taste profile similar to sucrose, are stable at pH values above 3 and at temperatures up to 140°C (37). Since fructo-oligosaccharides are non-reducing oligosaccharides, they do not undergo the Maillard browning reaction.

Polysaccharides

Starch

Starch is the most important, abundant, digestible food polysaccharide. It occurs as the reserve polysaccharide in the leaf, stem (pith), root (tuber), seed, fruit and pollen of many higher plants. It occurs as discrete, partially-crystalline granules whose size, shape, and gelatinization temperature depend on the botanical source of the starch. Common food starches are derived from seed (wheat, maize, rice, barley) and root (potato, cassava/tapioca) sources (see Table 6). Starches have been modified to improve desired functional characteristics and are added in relatively small amounts to foods as food additives.

Starch is a homopolysaccharide composed only of glucose units and consists of a mixture of two polymers, amylose and amylopectin, whose glucopyranosyl units are linked almost entirely through α-D-(1->4)-glucosidic bonds. Amylose shows many of the properties of a linear polymer and has historically been considered to be a linear polymer with a degree of polymerization of approximately 1000 or less. However, it is now known that amylose contains a limited amount of branching involving α-D-(1->6)-glucosidic linkages at the branch points. Amylopectin is a high molecular weight, highly branched polymer containing about 5-6% of α-D-(1->6)-glucosidic linkages as the branch points. The average chain length is 20 to 25 units with an average degree of polymerization in the thousands, and molecular weight in the millions.

While the manner in which amylose and amylopectin are organized to form the starch granule is not clearly understood, the granule is partially crystalline exhibiting an x-ray diffraction pattern and birefringence. Most common cereal starches contain 20-30% amylose. Waxy starches (maize, rice, sorghum, barley) have no amylose and contain essentially 100% amylopectin. The first example of a waxy wheat starch has recently been reported from Japan. High-amylose starches (maize, barley) having 50-70% amylose are available. Waxy and high-amylose starches differ from normal starches in some properties that make them of use in certain food products. A number of double and triple maize starch mutants are being investigated to determine whether they have unique or desirable physicochemical and/or functional properties that would make them of use in selected food products.

TABLE 6
Some properties of whole granular starches

Source	Gelatinization Temperature Range, °C	Granule Shape	Granule Size (mm)	Iodine Binding Capacity (g I_2 / 100g)	Amylose Content (%)
Barley	51-60	Round or lenticular	20-25 2-6	4.3	22
Triticale	55-62	Round	19 (2-35)	-	23-24
Wheat	58-64	Lenticular or Round	20-35 2-10	5.0	26 (23-27)
Rye	57-70	Round or lenticular	28 (12-40)	5.5	27
Oats	53-59	Polyhedral	5-10	5.1	23-24
Potato	59-68	Oval	40 (15-100)	4.5	23
Maize	62-72	Round or polyhedral	15 (5-25)	5.3	28
Waxy maize	63-72	Round	15 (5-25)	0.1	1
Broad bean	64-67	Oval	30	4.5	24
Sorghum	68-78	Round	15-35	-	25 (23-28)
Rice	68-78	Polygonal	3-8		17-19* 21-22**
High amylose Maize	67-80	Round Irregular sausage shaped	25	ca. 10.5	52
Peas smooth	55/70	Reniform*** (simple)	5-10	6.7	33-36
wrinkled	>99	Reniform*** (cmpd)	30-40	14.7	71-76

* japonica; ** indica; *** kidney-shaped

Starch granules are not water soluble but easily hydrate in aqueous solution, swelling about 10% in volume. When an aqueous suspension of granules is heated, additional swelling occurs until a temperature is reached where there is a transition from organization to disorganization. This is known as the gelatinization temperature and normally occurs over a range of about 10°C. The digestion of starch by α-amylase is greatly enhanced by gelatinization. Upon further heating (pasting or cooking), swelling continues and the amylose and portions of the amylopectin leach from the granule producing a viscous suspension. Cooling of this suspension leads to the formation of a gel. With further time, realignment of the linear chains of amylose and the short chains of amylopectin can occur in the process known as retrogradation. In food products based on starch gels, this can lead to liquid being expressed from the gel in the phenomenon known as syneresis, which is generally an undesirable occurrence. Retrogradation is most rapid with amylose and much slower and more incomplete with amylopectin due to the short chain length of its branches.

Modified starches

Many starches do not have the functional properties needed to impart or maintain desired qualities in food products. As a result, some starches have been modified to obtain the functional properties required. The types of modified starches, also known as starch derivatives, and some of their functional properties are listed in Table 7 (38).

The starches most commonly modified for commercial use are those from normal maize, tapioca, potato, and waxy maize. Modified starches are used to improve viscosity, shelf stability, particulate integrity, processing parameters, textures, appearance and emulsification. While virtually all of the different types of modified starches find use in the food industry, substituted and cross-linked starches are particularly important. These two types of modified starches are produced by reactions in which a small number of hydroxyl groups on the glucose units of amylose and amylopectin, mostly in amorphous regions and on the surface of the granule, are modified without destroying the granular nature of the starch.

Substituted starches are produced by etherification or esterification. This reduces the tendency of chains to realign (retrograde) following gelatinization of starch during heat processing. Substitution lowers the gelatinization temperature, gives freeze-thaw stability, increases viscosity, increases clarity, inhibits gel formation, and reduces syneresis.

Cross-linked starches are produced by introducing a limited number of linkages between the chains of amylose and amylopectin using difunctional reagents. Cross-linking essentially reinforces the hydrogen bonding occurring within the granule. It increases gelatinization temperature; improves acid stability, heat stability and shear stability; inhibits gel formation; and controls viscosity during processing.

TABLE 7
Types of modified starches

Modified starch	Functional properties
Bleached	Oxidized - Lighten colour, sterilize
Converted	Hydrolyzed - Reduces viscosity
(a) Thin boiling	Fluidity
(b) Dextrins	Dry roasting
(c) Oxidized	Creaminess, short body
Crosslinked	Strengthens granule
	Increases viscosity
	Tolerance to acidity
	Yields shear to resistance
	Heat penetration
Stabilized	Resist retrogradation
	Low temperature stability

Dietary fibre

Dietary fibre has been considered to be composed of non-starch polysaccharides plus lignin plus resistant oligosaccharides plus resistant starch. Since lignin is not a carbohydrate, it will not be discussed. Dietary fibre occurring in foods and food products can be considered to consist of cellulose, hemicelluloses, pectic substances, hydrocolloids (gums and mucilages), resistant starches, and resistant oligosaccharides.

Cellulose, the major cell wall structural component in plants, is an unbranched linear chain of several thousand glucose units with β-D-(1->4)-glucosidic linkages. Cellulose's mechanical strength, resistance to biological degradation, low aqueous solubility, and resistance to acid hydrolysis result from hydrogen bonding within the microfibrils (39). There is a portion (10-15%) of the total cellulose, referred to as "amorphous," that is more readily acid hydrolyzed. Controlled acid hydrolysis of the amorphous fraction yields microcrystalline cellulose. Cellulose has been used as a bulking agent in food due to its water-absorbing ability and low solubility. Some of the early dietary fibre ingredient sources were based on cellulose powders or microcrystalline cellulose. Cellulose is not digested to any extent by the enzymes of the human gastrointestinal system.

Hemicelluloses may be present in soluble and insoluble forms and are comprised of a number of branched and linear pentose- and hexose-containing polysaccharides. In cereal grains, soluble hemicelluloses are termed "pentosans." Hemicelluloses are of much lower molecular weight than cellulose. Component monosaccharide units may include xylose, arabinose, galactose, mannose, glucose, glucuronic acid, and galacturonic acid.

Mixed linkage β-glucans, the (1->3)(1->4)-β-D-glucans, have generated considerable interest in recent years due to their physiological response as soluble dietary fibre. While these glucans are found in relatively small quantities in wheat, they are a major component of cell-call material in barley and oats. These glucans form viscous aqueous solutions and have been shown to be effective in reducing serum cholesterol concentrations (40). Oat bran, a rich source of β-D-glucan, has been incorporated into many food products, particularly cereals, as a source of the soluble fibre that has been touted for cholesterol reduction.

Both soluble and insoluble hemicelluloses play important roles in food products, the former functioning as soluble and the latter as insoluble fibre. They are characterized by their ability to bind water and hence serve as bulking agents. The presence of acidic components in some hemicelluloses impart the capacity to bind cations. Hemicelluloses are fermented to a greater extent than cellulose in the colon.

Pectins find widespread use in foods such as jams and jellies because of their ability to form stable gels. Completely esterified pectins do not require the addition of acid or electrolyte to form gels. The presence of calcium salts enhances the gelling capacity and decreases the dependence on pH and sugar concentration. Pectic substances are of importance as a component of dietary fibre because of their ion-exchange properties, due to the presence of the galacturonic acid units, and gelling (viscosity enhancing) properties.

Hydrocolloids (gums, mucilages) are used in small amounts in food products for their thickening (viscosity increasing), gelling, stabilizing, or emulsifying ability. They are derived from seaweed extracts, plant exudates, seeds, and microbial sources.

Resistant starch

While starch was long thought to be completely digested, it is now recognized that there is a portion (resistant starch) which resists digestion, passes into the lower intestine, and is fermented there. Resistant starch has been defined as "the sum of starch and products of starch degradation not absorbed in the small intestine of healthy individuals" (41). Three types of resistant starch have been identified (41,42):

1. RS1 - Physically trapped starch: These starch granules are physically trapped within a food matrix so that digestive enzymes are prevented or delayed from having access to them. This can occur in whole or partly ground grains, seeds, cereals, and legumes. The amount of type 1 resistant starch will be affected by food processing and can be decreased or eliminated by milling.

2. RS2 - Resistant starch granules: Certain raw (native) starch granules, such as potato and green banana, are known to resist attack by α-amylase. This is probably related to the crystalline nature of the starch (i.e., crystalline regions of the starch granule are less susceptible to attack by acid and enzymes than the amorphous regions). Gelatinization normally occurs during cooking and food processing, although the extent is dependent on the moisture content of the food product and may not be complete in water-limited systems (e.g. sugar cookies). Gelatinized starch is much more rapidly digested by enzymes than is raw starch. Gelatinized potato and green banana starch are digested by α-amylases.

High-amylose maize starches have high gelatinization temperatures, requiring temperatures that are often not reached in conventional cooking practices (154-171°C) before the granules are completely disrupted. As a result, undigested starch granules have been observed in the effluent from ileostomates fed a meal containing high amylose maize (41). These starches offer an opportunity to manipulate the amount of resistant starch present in food products.

3. <u>RS3 - Retrograded starch</u>: The amylose and amylopectin components of starch undergo the process of retrogradation in a time dependent process after starch has been gelatinized/cooked. The rate at which amylose retrogrades is much higher than that for amylopectin which has much shorter chain lengths. Amylose can be retrograded to a form that resists dispersion in water and digestion with α-amylase (41). This form of resistant starch can be generated during food processing.

    There is currently great interest in resistant starch because of is potential use as a food ingredient to increase the dietary fibre content of foods and also because it may be possible to manipulate the amount of resistant starch in food products through processing conditions.

Sugar alcohols (alditols, polyols)

Monosaccharides and disaccharides in which the aldose and ketose functional groups have been reduced to hydroxyl groups are known as sugar alcohols (alditols, polyols). Sugar alcohols, such as sorbitol, occur in small amounts in fruits. Due to their physicochemical properties and relative sweetness, sugar alcohols have found use as bulk sweeteners. Xylitol has a negative heat of solubility which produces a cooling sensation when used in products such as chewing gum. The sugar alcohols undergo limited absorption in the small intestine, and this can lead to laxative effects in many people when large amounts (50 grams or more at one time) are consumed. There appear to be no other health risks associated with the consumption of sugar alcohols.

DIETARY FIBRE AND RESISTANT STARCH ANALYSIS

Dietary fibre

There is no single analytical method which meets all the requirements for the nutritional or chemical components of dietary fibre in foods. Analytical methods and techniques continue to be improved, whether this results from changes in the purposes of the analysis or improvements in the accuracy, precision, rapidity, ruggedness and cost effectiveness of the method. This subject has been recently reviewed (43,44).

Currently, dietary fibre methodology can be classified into three major categories as follows:

1. Nonenzymatic-gravimetric
2. Enzymatic-gravimetric
3. Enzymatic-chemical methods, which include
   a. Enzymatic-colorimetric
   b. Enzymatic-GLC/HPLC

For most foods, the older nonenzymatic-gravimetric methods do not recover a significant portion of what is considered to be total dietary fibre. Among those, the crude fibre method measures fibre as the sum of lignin and cellulose, the acid detergent method measures fibre as the sum of lignin, cellulose, and acid insoluble hemicellulose, and the neutral detergent method measures fibre as the sum of lignin, cellulose and neutral detergent insoluble hemicellulose.

The realization that neither the crude fibre nor the neutral and acid detergent fibre methods were satisfactory for measuring any of the soluble dietary fibre and some of the insoluble dietary fibre led researchers to explore enzymatic approaches for the determination of dietary fibre.

Enzymatic-gravimetric methods

In the early 1980s, a enzymatic-gravimetric method was developed in which the sum of soluble and insoluble polysaccharides and lignin were measured as a unit and considered to be total dietary fibre (TDF). That method is detailed in section 45.4.07 of the AOAC International Official Methods of Analysis (45). The procedure was later extended to the determination of insoluble dietary fibre (IDF) (32.1.16 AOAC) (45) and soluble dietary fibre (SDF) (45.4.08 AOAC) (45). All three methods use the same basic enzymatic-gravimetric procedure with phosphate buffer. An additional method to determine TDF, IDF and SDF was developed in the early 1990s and is detailed in 32.1.17 AOAC (45). It is similar to the first method, in that it uses the same three enzymes (heat stable α-amylase, protease, and amyloglucosidase) and similar incubation conditions but substitutes 2-(N-morpholino) ethanesulfonic acid-tris (hydroxymethyl) aminomethane (MES-TRIS) buffer for the phosphate buffer. The results using the MES-TRIS buffer for determination of dietary fibre are similar to those obtained using the phosphate buffer. The analytical scheme for this procedure is summarized in Figure 4.

Figure 4

Analysis of Total Dietary Fibre (TDF), Insoluble Dietary Fibre (TDF) and Soluble Dietary Fibre (SDF) by AOAC method 32.1.17 (45)

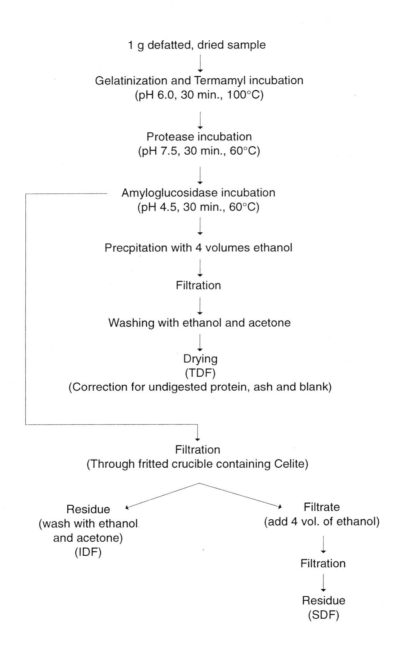

Source: Adapted from AOAC International 1995 (45)

Enzymatic-chemical methods

Another method recently accepted for official action by the AOAC for the determination of TDF is one based on assays for components of TDF - neutral sugars, uronic acid residues and Klason lignin (45.4.11 AOAC) (45). This procedure is often referred to as the Uppsala Method. Starch is removed enzymatically and soluble polymers are precipitated with ethanol. Precipitated and insoluble polysaccharides are hydrolyzed using sulfuric acid and the released neutral sugars are quantitated as alditol acetates using gas-liquid chromatography. Uronic acids in the acid hydrolysate are determined by colorimetry. Klason lignin is determined gravimetrically. The three values are added together to obtain the TDF figure.

Plant cell wall material comprises much of what is considered to be fibre in the diet. About 90% of endogenous plant cell wall material consists of non-starch polysaccharides (NSP) (46). The analytical procedure known as the Englyst method determines NSP after enzymatic removal of starch, precipitation of NSP, followed by acid hydrolysis and measurement of the released constituent sugars. In an early method the sugars were assayed colourimetrically (47) and in a more recent procedure, they are quantitated by any of three instrumental techniques, i.e. gas-liquid chromatography, high performance liquid chromatography and colourimetry (48).

Resistant starch

Of the many analytical procedures employed for resistant starch (RS), two have emerged as the leading candidates for approval. These are the methods described by Englyst (49) and Champ (50). They both provide similar results. The first step is removal of digestible starch from the food sample using pancreatic α-amylase (in cases where there may be inhibition of the pancreatic enzyme by products of digestion, amyloglucosidase is added). Sometimes the amylolysis is preceded by a proteolysis step with pepsin and trypsin to mimic the action of the stomach and intestine. The RS is quantitated either directly in the residue (50) or by difference between total starch and digestible starch, which are determined separately (49).

A new procedure has been proposed which is derived from several RS analysis systems (51). Its principle is that *in-vitro* RS is defined as that starch which is not hydrolyzed by incubation with α-amylase. Amyloglucosidase is added to avoid inhibition by by-products of amylase digestion. Hydrolysis products are extracted with 80% ethanol and discarded. The RS is then solubilized with 2N potassium hydroxide and hydrolyzed with amyloglucosidase. The procedure is relatively simple with no particular training required, and is summarized in Figure 5.

Figure 5

Method for the determination of resistant starch

100 mg sample*
Add 10 ml enzyme solution in buffer (pH 6.9); pancreatic α-amylase (500U);
0.1M tris-maleate buffer solution (calcium chloride 4mM)

↓

Mix 16 hours at 37°C; then add 40 ml ethanol

↓

Leave 1 hour; then centrifuge

↓

Wash residue twice with 80% EtOH, dry at 60°C
Add 1.56 ml H_2O, then add 1.5 ml 4M KOH

↓

Mix 0.5 hours at room temperature
Add 12 ml H2O

↓

To 1.5 ml dispersion, add approximately 0.65 ml 2M acetic acid (to obtain pH 4.5)
and 0.1 ml amyloglucosidase (20U/0.1 ml 0.1M Na acetate buffer pH 4.5)
Shake 90 min. at 65°C

↓

Determine glucose using glucose oxidase assay
The result is resistant starch

* Ground in a mincer. The sample must be weighed to contain 50 mg starch
Source: Adapted from Champ, M., Noah, L., Loizeau, G., Kozlowski, F. (51)

EFFECTS OF FOOD PROCESSING ON DIETARY CARBOHYDRATES

Introduction

Dietary guidelines for developed countries are consistent in recommending an increased carbohydrate intake, corresponding to at least 55% of total energy. Correspondingly, the carbohydrate content in diets typical for developing countries should be maintained at a high level. The nutritional quality of the carbohydrates and the effects of processing on that quality then becomes a concern, because both the content and the nutritional quality of food carbohydrates can be altered by processing in a number of ways.

Carbohydrate loss through leaching

Low molecular weight carbohydrates

During wet heat treatment, as in blanching, boiling and canning of vegetables and fruits, there is a considerable loss of low molecular weight carbohydrates (i.e. mono- and disaccharides) as well as micronutrients, into the processing water. For example, in the blanching of carrots and swedes (rutabagas) there was a loss of 25% and 30%, respectively of these carbohydrates. With subsequent boiling another 20% was lost. In peas, green beans and Brussels sprouts the loss was less pronounced — about 12% following blanching and another 7-13% at boiling (52).

The loss of glucose and fructose at boiling was higher than that of sucrose (53). The losses of low molecular weight carbohydrates in carrots have also been shown to differ between various cultivars, and also to be different at harvest and in storage. After storage the loss of low molecular weight carbohydrates increases following boiling, most probably due to the higher water content and therefore also a higher diffusitivity (54). The loss of low molecular weight carbohydrates, at least in carrots, seems to be relatively easy to predict by knowing initial concentrations and process conditions of the raw material.

Dietary fibre

No leaching of dietary fibre into the processing water has been reported with blanching, boiling and canning of carrots, green peas, green beans and Brussels sprouts (52). With swedes, however, there was a 40% loss of dietary fibre (mainly insoluble) with boiling. Also with canning there was a leakage of insoluble fibre into the processing water.

Alterations of low molecular weight carbohydrates

Production of resistant oligosaccharides

The production of resistant oligosaccharides by enzyme technology is an expanding area. More than half of the "functional foods" on the Japanese market contain prebiotic oligosaccharides as active component, with the aim of promoting favourable gut microflora. Fructo-oligosaccharides synthesized from sucrose (55) and galacto-oligosaccharides synthesized from lactose are the most extensively used types of resistant oligosaccharides. Alternatively, fructo-oligosaccharides can be produced by hydrolysis of inulin.

Maillard reactions

Non-enzymatic browning reactions (Maillard reactions) occur between reducing sugars and amino groups in foods at processing and in storage. These reactions are temperature dependent and most extensive at intermediate water activities. They are important nutritionally as they may diminish the bioavailability of amino acids, especially lysine, thus diminishing the protein nutritional value. The carbohydrate content and availability is influenced only marginally.

When a non-reducing disaccharide such as sucrose is replaced by, for example, high fructose corn syrup containing glucose and fructose, Maillard reactions occur much more rapidly and extensively. This has to be kept in mind in selecting processing procedures and storage conditions.

Starch - heat-induced effects

Gelatinization

Gelatinization refers to the irreversible loss of the crystalline regions in starch granules that occur upon heating in the presence of water. The temperature range during which the crystalline structure of the starch granule is lost is dependent on the water content, and on the type of starch. The gelatinization dramatically increases the availability of starch for digestion by amylolytic enzymes.

Usually, the starch granules are not completely dissolved during food processing, and a food can be regarded as a dispersion in which starch granules and/or granular remnants constitute the dispersed phase. The degree of gelatinization achieved by most commonly used food processes, however, is sufficient to permit the starch to be rapidly digested. Consequently, even food processes which result in a low degree of gelatinization (e.g. steaming and flaking of cereals), produces a postprandial blood glucose and insulin increment similar to that with completely gelatinized foods (56,57).

Retrogradation

Gelatinized starch is not in thermodynamic equilibrium. There is, therefore, a progressive re-association of the starch molecules upon ageing (58). This recrystallization is referred to as retrogradation, and may reduce the digestibility of the starch. The retrogradation of the amylopectin component is a long-term phenomena occurring gradually upon storage of starchy foods. Amylose, however, re-associates more quickly. The crystallinity of retrograded amylopectin is lost following re-heating to approximately 70°C, whereas temperatures above 145°C are required to remove crystallinity of retrograded amylose. This is a temperature well above the range used for processing of starchy foods. This implies that retrograded amylose, once formed, will retain its crystallinity following re-heating of the food.

Par-boiling

During par-boiling of rice, the kernels are subjected to a pre-treatment involving heating and drying. This process reduces the stickiness of the rice, possibly by allowing leached amylose to retrograde and/or form inclusion complexes with polar lipids on the kernel surface. Par-boiling also affects the final cooking properties of the rice.

Starch -texturization

In pasta products, gluten forms a viscoelastic network that surrounds the starch granules, which restricts swelling and leaching during boiling. Pasta extrusion is known to result in products where the starch is slowly digested and absorbed (59,60). Available data on spaghetti also suggest that this product group is a comparatively rich source of resistant starch (61). The slow-release features of starch in pasta probably relates to the continuous glutenous phase. This not only restricts swelling, but possibly also results in a more gradual release of the starch substrate for enzymatic digestion. Pasta is now generally acknowledged as a low glycemic index food suitable in the diabetic diet. However, it should be noted that canning of pasta importantly increases the enzymic availability of starch, and hence the glycemic response (62).

Dietary fibre

Milling and peeling

During milling of cereal grains to refined flours the outer fibre-rich layers are removed, resulting in a lower content of total dietary fibre. This reduction is due mainly to a decrease of insoluble fibre. The dietary fibre composition in both whole-grain and refined flours is different. Refined flours of oats, barley, rice and sorghum contain mainly glucans, while arabinoxylans dominate in refined flours of wheat, rye and maize. Whole-grain flours all contain considerable amounts of cellulose. The husk which surrounds barley, rice and oats also contains considerable amounts of xylans. This fraction is generally removed before consumption, but oat and rice husks are used for fibre preparation to enrich foods.

Heat-treatment

Processes involving heat-treatment may affect the dietary fibre in different ways. An increased temperature leads to a breakage of weak bonds between polysaccharide chains. Also glycosidic linkages in the dietary fibre polysaccharides may be broken. These changes are important from analytical, functional and nutritional points of view.

A decreased association between fibre molecules, and/or a depolymerization of the fibre, results in a solubilization. If the depolymerization is extensive, alcohol soluble fragments can be formed, resulting in a decreased content of dietary fibre with many of the currently used fibre methods. Moderate depolymerization and/or decreased association between fibre molecules, may have only minor influence on the dietary fibre content, but functional (e.g. viscosity and hydration) and physiological properties of the fibre will be changed. Other reactions during processing that may affect the dietary fibre content and its properties are leakage into the processing water, formation of Maillard reaction products thus adding to the lignin content, and formation of resistant starch fractions. Also structural alterations in the cell wall architecture are important to follow during processing as these are highly correlated to sensory and nutritional characteristics.

The architecture of the fibre matrix in the cell wall differs between various types of plant material. The cross-linking of constituent polysaccharides and phenolics within the cell wall is important in determining the properties of the fibre matrix, as the solubility of the fibre is highly dependent on the type and amount of cross-links present. During heat-treatment the cell-wall matrix is modified and the structural alterations that occur may be important not only for the nutritional properties of the product but also for its palatability.

With extrusion-cooking of wheat-flour, even at mild conditions, the solubility of the dietary fibre increases (63). The solubilization seems to be dependent on the water content used in the process, and the lower the content of water, the higher the solubilization of the fibre, at least for whole-grain wheat flour and wheat bran (64). The screw speed and the temperature had minor effects in those experiments. An increased solubility of the fibre has also been obtained with 'severe' popping of wheat (52), whereas baking (conventional and sour-dough baking), steam-flaking and drum-drying had only minor effects on dietary fibre components (65). One reason why popping caused an increased solubility of the fibre was that the outer fibrous layers were removed and the content of insoluble fibre decreased. Considerable amounts of Maillard reaction products were also formed during this process. A loss of insoluble dietary fibre has also been reported with autoclaving of wheat flour, which was attributed to degradation of the arabinoxylans (65).

Hydration properties (swelling, water-holding and water-binding capacity)

Most raw materials containing cereal fibres are ground for better acceptance of the final product and this process can affect hydration properties. Swelling and water-binding capacity of pea hull fibres are decreased by grinding, whereas the water-holding capacity was slightly increased (66). The kinetics of water-uptake was also different, and the ground product hydrated instantaneously in contrast to the unground product, which reached equilibrium only after 30 minutes. This was related to the differences in surface area.

Heat-treatment can also change hydration properties. For example, boiling increased the water-binding capacity slightly in wheat bran and apple fibre products, whereas autoclaving, steam-cooking and roasting had no significant effects (67). The kinetics of water uptake, however, was different for steam-cooking and roasting. Thus, both products exposed to steam-cooking had a very rapid water-uptake, whereas the roasted sample had a slow uptake. Extrusion-cooking of pea-hulls, sugar-beet fibres, wheat bran and lemon fibres had only slight effects on the water-binding capacity.

Summary

Processing of foods affects carbohydrate and micronutrient content and bioavailability in different ways with either desirable or adverse effects on the nutritional value. Losses of water-soluble nutrients at blanching and boiling can be minimized by use of small amounts of water and by adding back the processing water.

The bioavailability of starch is affected dramatically through processing, regarding both rate and extent of small-intestinal digestibility. This permits optimizing the digestion of starch by choice of raw materials and processing conditions.

Processing effects on dietary fibre include solubilization and depolymerization, that can influence physiological effects both in the upper and lower gastrointestinal tract. Formation of resistant starch and use of resistant oligosaccharides as food ingredients provide new opportunities to increase the amount of carbohydrate available for colonic fermentation.

DIGESTION, ABSORPTION AND ENERGY VALUE OF CARBOHYDRATES

Introduction

Much has been learned about carbohydrate digestion and absorption over the last 20 years, and this new knowledge has, in many ways, changed completely the way we think about dietary carbohydrates. We now know that starches are not completely digested, and, indeed, some are quite poorly digested. We have learned that the undigestible carbohydrates are not just neutral bulking agents, but have important physiologic effects, and even contribute energy to the diet. "Sugar" is not bad for health, and starches are not all equal in their effects on blood glucose and lipids. However, knowledge in all these areas is far from complete. In addition, there is unresolved controversy about how to define and how to measure dietary fibre and starch, and different methods are in use in different parts of the world. This presents a major challenge for those who have the responsibility of formulating policies and recommendations about dietary carbohydrates and how the energy value and carbohydrate composition of foods is determined.

Energy value of carbohydrates

Many different methods have been used to determine how much of the energy in foods is available for human metabolism, termed metabolizable energy (ME). The total amount of energy in a food (TE) can be determined by calorimetry, but ME is less than TE because not all the energy in food is absorbed and some is absorbed, but lost in the urine. Most of the energy not absorbed ends in the feces, but some is lost in the gases and heat produced during colonic fermentation.

The most common approach for determining the energy content of foods is the factorial method (68) in which the amount of energy contained in each of the various components of the food (ie. fat, protein, carbohydrate, alcohol) is calculated, and the sum of the resulting figures is taken as the amount of energy in the food. Determining the energy value of carbohydrate presents a conceptual challenge because carbohydrates vary in their gross energy content per gram, the degree to which they are digested and absorbed, and the fact that the undigestible carbohydrates provide an amount of energy which depends upon the degree to which they are fermented in the colon. This may vary from 0 to 100%. Alternative empirical models have been proposed based on regression equations developed from experiments where gross energy intake and energy excretion in urine and stool were measured on a variety of diets. Here, metabolizable energy in the diet is equal to gross energy intake minus energy losses, the latter being estimated from nitrogen and unavailable carbohydrate intakes. It has been argued that empirical models for determining the energy content of the diet are more accurate than the factorial approach because they have fewer and smaller sources of error (68). Nevertheless, it seems unlikely that the factorial approach will be replaced, at least in the near future, because it is ingrained in food labelling regulations and food tables.

Digestion and absorption of carbohydrates

Polysaccharides and oligosaccharides must be hydrolyzed to their component monosaccharides before being absorbed. The digestion of starch begins with salivary amylase, but this activity is much less important than that of pancreatic amylase in the small intestine. Amylase hydrolyzes starch, with the primary end products being maltose, maltotriose, and α-dextrins, although some glucose is also produced. The products of α-amylase digestion are hydrolyzed into their component monosaccharides by enzymes expressed on the brush border of the small intestinal cells, the most important of which are maltase, sucrase, isomaltase and lactase (69). With typical refined Western diets, carbohydrate digestion is rapid and carbohydrate absorption occurs primarily in the upper small intestine. This is reflected by the presence of finger-like villi in the mucosa of the upper small intestine, with wider and shorter villi in the lower half of the small intestine. However, carbohydrate digestion and absorption can occur along the entire length of the small intestine, and is shifted toward the ileum when the diet contains less readily digested carbohydrates, or when intestinal glucosidase inhibitors which may be used to treat diabetes are present. In this situation, the upper small intestine exhibits wide villous structures with leaf-like arrays, while in the ileum the villi become longer and more finger-like.

Monosaccharides

Only D-glucose and D-galactose are actively absorbed in the human small intestine. D-fructose is not actively absorbed, but has a rate of diffusion greater than would be expected by passive diffusion. The sodium dependent glucose transporter, SGLT1, is responsible for the active transport of glucose or galactose with an equimolar amount of sodium against a concentration gradient into the cytoplasm of the enterocyte. Fructose is taken up by facilitated transport by the glucose transporter 5 (GLUT5). Glucose is pumped out of the enterocyte into the intracellular space by the glucose transporter 2 (GLUT2) (70). The complete mechanism of fructose absorption in the human intestine is not understood. When fructose is given alone in solution, 40-80% of subjects have malabsorption, and some subjects can absorb less than 15g fructose. Flatulence and diarrhoea are common if doses of fructose over 50g are given by mouth. However, if fructose is given in combination with glucose or starch, fructose is completely absorbed, even in subjects who malabsorb fructose alone (71). Since fructose rarely occurs in the diet in the absence of other carbohydrates, fructose malabsorption is really only a problem for studies involving oral fructose loads.

Disaccharides

Intestinal brush border glucosidases tend to be inducible. For example, there is evidence that a high sucrose intake increases the postprandial insulin and the gastric inhibitory polypeptide responses to large loads of oral sucrose (72), which probably reflects an increased rate of absorption due to induction of intestinal sucrase activity. Lack of brush border glucosidases results in an inability to absorb specific carbohydrates. This occurs rarely, except for lactase deficiency which is common in non-Caucasian populations. The latter may be complete or partial and results in a reduced ability to digest and absorb lactose.

The Glycemic Index

The blood glucose responses of carbohydrate foods can be classified by the glycemic index (GI). The GI is considered to be a valid index of the biological value of dietary carbohydrates. It is defined as the glycemic response elicited by a 50g carbohydrate portion of a food expressed as a percent of that elicited by a 50g carbohydrate portion of a standard food (73). The glycemic response is defined as the incremental area under the blood glucose response curve, ignoring the area beneath the fasting concentration (i.e. the area beneath the curve) (74-76). The standard food has been glucose or white bread. If glucose is the standard, (ie. GI of glucose = 100) the GI values of foods are lower than if white bread is the standard by a factor of 1.38 because the glycemic response of glucose is 1.38 times that of white bread. GI values for several hundred foods have been published (77,78) (see Table 8).

The Glycemic Index and Mixed Meals

The validity of the GI has been the subject of much controversy, mostly because of supposed lack of application to mixed meals. Much of the controversy has been because of application of inappropriate methods to estimate the expected glycemic responses for mixed meals. When properly applied, the GI predicts, with reasonable accuracy, the relative blood glucose responses of mixed meals of the same composition but consisting of different carbohydrate foods (79).

Implications of the Glycemic Index

There are a number of long-term implications of altering the rate of absorption, or GI, of dietary carbohydrate. There is good evidence that reducing diet GI improves overall blood glucose control in subjects with diabetes (80) and reduces serum triglycerides in subjects with hypertriglyceridemia (81).

There is also some evidence that the glycemic index is relevant to sports nutrition and appetite regulation. Low GI foods eaten before prolonged strenuous exercise increased endurance time and provided higher concentrations of plasma fuels toward the end of exercise (82). However, high GI foods led to faster replenishment of muscle glycogen after exercise (83).

TABLE 8
Glycemic index of selected foods (continues on next page)

	GI*	n**		GI*	n**
BAKED GOODS			**GRAINS**		
Cakes	87±5	9	Pearled barley	36±3	4
Cookies	90±3	14	Cracked barley	72	1
Crackers, wheat	99±4	8	Buckwheat	78±6	3
Muffins	88±9	8	Bulgur	68±3	4
Rice cakes	123±6	2	Couscous	93±9	2
			Cornmeal	98±1	3
BREADS					
Barley kernel	49±5	3	Sweet corn	78±2	7
Barley flour	95±2	2	Millet	101	1
Rye kernel	71±3	6	Rice, white	81±3	13
Rye flour	92±3	10	Rice, low amylose	126±4	3
Rye crispbread	93±2	5	Rice, high amylose	83±5	3
White bread	101±0	5	Rice, brown	79±6	3
Whole-meal flour	99±3	12	Rice, instant	128±4	2
Other products[a]	100±4	5	Rice, parboiled	68±4	13
			Specialty rices	78±2	5
BREAKFAST CEREALS			Rye kernels	48±4	3
All bran	60±7	4	Tapioca	115±9	1
Cornflakes	119±5	4	Wheat keenelsa	59±4	4
Muesli	80±14	4			
Oat bran	78±8	2	**DAIRY PRODUCTS**		
Porridge oats	87±2	8	Ice cream	84±9	6
Puffed rice	123±11	3	Milk, whole	39±9	4
Puffed wheat	105±3	2	Milk, skim	46	1
Shredded wheat	99±9	3	Yogurt[d]	48±1	2
Other, GI≥80[b]	103±3	15	Yogurt[e]	27±7	2
Other, GI<80[c]	72±2	4			
FRUIT			**LEGUMES**		
Apple	52±3	4	Baked beans	69±12	2
Apple juice	58±1	2	Black-eyed peas	59±12	2
Apricots, dried	44±2	2	Butter beans	44±3	3
Apricots, canned	91	1	Chickpeas	47±2	3
Banana	83±6	5	Canned chickpeas	59±1	2
Banana, underripe	51±8	2	Haricot beans	54±8	5
Banana, overripe	82±8	2	Kidney beans	42±6	7
Kiwifruit	75±8	2	Kidney beans, canned	74	1
Mango	80±7	2	Lentils	38±3	6
Orange	62±6	4	Lentils, green	42±6	3
Orange juice	74±4	3	Lentils, green canned	74	1
Paw paw	83±3	2	Lima beans	46	1
Peach, canned	67±12	3	Peas, dried green	56±12	2
Pear	54±4	4	Peas, green	68±7	3
Other, GI<80[f]	54±7	7	Pinto beans	61±3	3
Other, GI≥80[g]	92±4	5	Soya beans	23±3	3
			Split peas, yellow	45	1

TABLE 8
Glycemic index of selected foods (continued)

	GI*	n**		GI*	n**
PASTA			**SNACKS**		
Linguine	71±4	6	Jelly beans	114	1
Macaroni	64	1	Lifesavers	100	1
Macaroni, boxed	92	1	Chocolate (various)	84±14	2
Spaghetti, white	59±4	10	Popcorn	79	1
Spaghetti, durum	78±7	3	Corn chips	105±2	2
Spaghetti, brown	53±7	2	Potato chips	77±4	2
Other	59±3	8	Peanuts	21±12	3
POTATOES			**SOUPS**		
Instant	118±2	5	Bean soups (various)	84±7	4
Baked	121±16	4	Tomato	54	1
New	81±8	3	**SUGARS**		
White, boiled	80±2	3	Honey	104±21	2
White, mashed	100±2	3	Fructose	32±2	4
French fries	107	1	Glucose	138±4	8
Sweet potato	77±11	2	Sucrose	87±2	5
Yam	73	1	Lactose	65±4	2

*GI=glycemic index (white bread=100), mean±SEM of mean values from various studies.
**Number of studies.

a Bagel, stuffing mix, hamburger bun, rolls, melba toast.

b Bran buds, Bran chex, Cheerios, Corn bran, Corn chex, Cream of wheat, Crispix, Golden Grahams, Grapenuts, Grapenuts flakes, Life, Pro stars, Sustain, Team, Total (GI range, 83-127)

c Bran buds with psyllium, Red River, Special K (Australia), Sultana bran (Australia) (GI range 67-77)

d Sweetened with sugar

e Artificially sweetened

f Cherries, fruit cocktail, grapefruit, grapefruit juice, grapes, plum, pineapple juice

g Pineapple, raisins, rockmelon, sultanas, watermelon

PHYSIOLOGICAL EFFECTS OF DIETARY FIBRE

Introduction

Although a great deal of research was stimulated throughout the world by the Burkitt and Trowell's hypothesis (84), it is still early to assign clear health claims to dietary fibre. This difficulty is due in great part to the fact that dietary fibre includes many complex substances, each having unique chemical structure and physical properties. Moreover, dietary fibre is often intimately associated in the plant cell structure with other organic compounds, such as vitamins, phyto-oestrogens, flavonoids, etc., displaying their own biological activity. Nevertheless, numerous prospective and well-designed experimental studies have highlighted several physiological and metabolic effects of dietary fibre which may be important for human health.

Digestive fate of dietary fibre

It is now well-established that dietary fibre reaches the large intestine and is fermented by the colonic microflora with the production of short chain fatty acids (SCFA), hydrogen, carbon dioxide and biomass. This fermentative process dominates human large bowel function and provides a means whereby energy is obtained from carbohydrates not digested in the small bowel, through absorption of SCFA.

Fermentation of fibre in the colon

Polysaccharides cannot penetrate in the bacterial cells. They are first hydrolysed in monosaccharides, by membranous or extra-cellular enzymes secreted by bacteria. Metabolism of these monomeric sugars continue in the bacterial cells using the Embden-Meyerhoff pathway which leads to pyruvate. Pyruvate does not appear in the large bowel because it is immediately converted in end-products. These are SCFA, mainly acetate, propionate and butyrate, and gases: carbon dioxide (CO_2), hydrogen (H_2), and methane (CH_4).

Colonic fermentation is an efficient digestive process since starch is almost totally degraded, as well as lactose, alcohol-sugars and fructans if the intake of these sugars is not too high. More than half of the usually consumed fibres are degraded in the large intestine, the rest being excreted in the stool (see Table 9). A number of factors are likely to affect the utilization of fermentable carbohydrates in the colon. Among these is solubility. The more soluble substrates, being more accessible to hydrolytic enzymes, are likely to be degraded more rapidly. Nevertheless, some soluble fibres such as alginates or carragheenans are poorly fermented. Other factors involving digestive motility and individual differences in microflora could also modulate fermentation. Furthermore, certain metabolic pathways can be modified by the repeated occurrence of some sugars (lactose, lactulose, fructans) in the colon. The mechanisms and the physiological consequences of this adaptation are not completely identified.

TABLE 9
Colonic fermentability of dietary fibres in humans

Dietary fibre	Fermentability (%)
Cellulose	20 - 80
Hemicelluloses	60 - 90
Pectins	100
Guar gum	100
Ispaghula	55
Wheat bran	50
Resistant starch	100
Inulin, oligosaccharides	100 (if they are not in excess)

Absorption and metabolism of end-products

Reducing the rate of digestion of carbohydrate spreads the absorption of carbohydrate along a longer portion of the small intestine (159,160), and tends to increase the amount of carbohydrate which escapes digestion in the small intestine (161). For example, the amount of carbohydrate from lentils entering the colon is 2.5 times as great as carbohydrate from bread. Increasing the delivery of starch to the colon has many implications which include those on the health of the colon itself and on systemic metabolism. It is believed that starch entering the colon is completely and rapidly fermented, mostly in the cecum (162). The fermentation of starch produces relatively more butyrate than the fermentation of dietary fibre (162), and resistant starch produces somewhat different fermentation products than readily digested starch (163).

A part of the products of fermentation are utilized by bacteria yielding energy and carbon necessary for synthesis and growth of the flora. Another part is eliminated in the stool or rectal gases, but the major part is absorbed by the colonic mucosa. Absorption of SCFA is rapid and leads to accumulation of bicarbonates and increase of pH in the lumen. Butyrate is considered to be the primary nutrient for the epithelial cells lining the colon (164), and SCFA stimulate proliferation of colonic epithelial cells and growth of the colon in general (165). Butyrate is the preferred substrate of colonocytes. SCFA which are not metabolized in the mucosa are oxidized in the liver, a part of acetate being also metabolised in the peripheric tissues.

Only a fraction of gases produced during fermentation is available for absorption. Hydrogen and methane are excreted in the breath gases. A large part of gases are consumed in the colonic lumen by bacteria. Acetogenic bacteria produce acetate from CO_2 and H_2. Methanogenic bacteria produce CH_4 by reduction of CO_2 with H_2. Finally, sulfate reducing bacteria utilise H_2 to reduce sulfates and produce sulfites or hydrogen sulfide. Unused gases are excreted through the anus.

Effects of dietary fibre on gut microflora

The composition of microflora appears to be influenced to some degree by diet, age and geographic considerations, but these factors are not thought to be particularly significant, at least as far as the commonly studied bacterial groups are concerned. Recent studies have shown, however, that the ingestion of certain oligosaccharides, such as fructo-oligosaccharides, could modify bacterial composition of the dominant flora by increasing bifidobacteria. Some studies suggest that these bifidobacteria, which are saccharolytic bacteria naturally occurring in the normal colonic flora, might be beneficial to host health. At the present time, however, this has not been conclusively established.

Ingestion of fructo-oligosaccharides have increased faecal counts of endogenous bifidobacteria by a factor of 10, without changing the total anaerobes concentration (85). The similarity of effects of chemically different substrates is likely due to the capacity of bifidobacteria to hydrolyze all these substrates and to metabolize the produced monomeric sugars (glucose, galactose, fructose). The exact mechanisms whereby only some substrates could stimulate preferentially the growth of bifidobactria are not known. A recent *in vitro* study suggested that the polymerization degree could be more determinant than the chemical nature of oligosaccharides (86). The metabolic consequences of the changes in faecal flora composition are unknown. Ingestion of oligosaccharides had no effect on stool weight and pH.

Effects of dietary fibre on gut function

In the gastrointestinal tract, some fibres form a matrix with fibrous characteristics. That is, some fibres, because of their ability to swell within the aqueous medium, can trap water and nutrients, especially water-soluble ones such as sugars. The physical characteristics of the gastric and small intestinal contents are altered by fibre sources. The bulk or amount of material in the gastrointestinal tract is greater because fibre is not digestible and hence remains during the transit of digesta through the small intestine. The volume increase is due to the water-holding capacity of certain fibres. The viscosity of the intestinal contents increases due to the presence of fibre sources containing viscous polysaccharides.

The changes in the physical characteristics of the intestinal contents may influence gastric emptying, dilute enzymes and absorbable compounds in the gut, prevent starch from hydrolyzing, and slow the diffusion or mobility of enzymes, substrates and nutrients to the absorptive surface. These effects result in the slower appearance of nutrients such as glucose and some lipid molecules in the plasma following a meal.

The effects of purified dietary fibres on bowel function may or may not be similar to those of intact fibres in whole foods. This is presumably due, at least in part, to interactions between fibre and starch, and the presence of fibre associated substances such as phytate and lectins which are present in the whole food. This makes it very difficult to make valid generalizations about the physiologic effects of fibre based simply on fibre analysis. For example, when considering the effect of fibre on postprandial blood glucose responses, purified viscous fibres have been found to produce a significant reduction in glycemic response in 33 of 50 studies (66%) reviewed in 1992, compared to only 3 of 14 (21%) studies with insoluble fibre (166). The effects of purified fibres appear to be directly related to their viscosity (167,168). This would suggest that the blood glucose responses of foods should be more closely related to their soluble than insoluble fibre content, however the opposite is the case. For 52 foods, the food glycemic index (as the indicator of rise in blood glucose) was weakly related to the amount of total fibre per 50g carbohydrate, and insoluble fibre explained a larger proportion of the variance in glycemic index, 17%, than soluble fibre, 9% (169).

Effects on carbohydrate digestion and absorption

Gastric emptying

Dietary fibres may affect gastric emptying in several ways (87). First, they may slow gastric filling, due to their bulking and energetic dilution capacity, which might in turn slow gastric emptying. Secondly, when certain soluble fibres are mixed in liquid meals or in liquid/solid meals, they delay emptying of gastric liquids by increasing viscosity of gastric contents. Such an increase in the viscosity of chyma could also slow the gastric emtying of solid components of the meal. On this issue, results are very controversial. Moreover, by acting as an emulsifier, viscous fibre can stabilize the gastric chyma and prevent separation of the solid from the liquid phase, impairing selective retention of the largest particles, and thereby increasing their rate of passage into the small intestine. Besides the effects of soluble fibres, insoluble fractions may also alter gastric emptying by mechanisms depending on their water retention capacity or size of particles.

Enzyme-substrate interaction

Available evidence suggests that fibre has little, if any, direct acute effect on the secretory function of the exocrine pancreas suggesting that the primary effect of fibre on carbohydrate digestion is exerted in the intestinal lumen. In the lumen, enzymes and substrates may be diluted with the addition of non-digestible material. Evidence from *in vitro* studies and from duodenal aspirates suggest that most of the tested fibres can alter the activity of pancreatic amylase (88). The inhibitory effects of fibre on pancreatic enzyme activities have been attributed to various factors including pH changes, ion-exchange properties, enzyme inhibitors and adsorption. Rather than a chemical enzyme-fibre interaction, the presence of fibre, through its particulate or viscous nature, probably impedes enzyme-substrate interaction.

The presence of fibre in a form that restricts starch gelatinization or access of the hydrolytic enzymes to starch can slow the rate of digestion of the starch. For instance, the slow rate of digestion of legumes may be related to the entrapment of starch in fibrous thick-walled cells, which prevents its complete swelling during cooking. In addition, resistance of starch to pancreatic hydrolysis may result from the presence of intact cell walls, which survive processing and cooking and insulate starch in such a manner that portions of it cannot be digested or absorbed.

Small intestinal motility

There is evidence that viscous fibres can influence accessibility of available carbohydrates to the mucosal surface and slow their absorption. One of the major mechanisms of this action is related to the effects of dietary fibre on small intestinal motility (89). Small intestinal contractions create turbulences and convective currents which cause fluid circulation and mixing of luminal contents. These movements allow glucose to be brought from the centre of the lumen close to the epithelium. When it reaches proximity to the epithelium, glucose must then diffuse across the unstirred water layer (UWL). This layer is created by a gradient of progressively poorer stirring as the mucosa is approached and forms an aqueous diffusion barrier separating mixed bulk luminal contents from the brush border. Thickness of the UWL depends on small intestinal contractions and is inversely related to the magnitude of the stir rate. When there is no contraction, fluid moves through the small intestine with laminar flow comparable to that occurring in a pipe. In this flow, there is no movement in the radial direction (from the centre of the lumen toward the epithelium), and consequently the stirring is very poor and the UWL very thick. On the contrary, normal motility generates both longitudinal and radial convection currents, hence creating turbulences and stirring of luminal fluid. Beside the effects of mixing contractions on glucose movement, small intestinal motility may alter absorption by influencing transit rate which determines area and time of contact between glucose and the epithelium.

Dietary fibres which alter small intestinal motility could thus influence glucose absorption by this mechanism. Viscous fibres, such as guar gum, stimulate motility but decrease transit rate, because they resist propulsive contractions. However, though guar gum slows transit it does not affect the distribution of glucose in the human upper small intestine. It is thus unlikely that guar gum delays glucose absorption by reducing contact area. As they resist propulsion, viscous fibres should similarly resist mixing contractions, hence inhibiting the effects of motility on fluid stirring. This is probably the mechanism by which they increase thickness of the UWL, and diminish passage of glucose across the epithelium.

Effects of dietary fibre on large bowel function

The major effects of dietary fibre occur in the colon. Here each type of dietary fibre interacts with the microflora, and the colonic mucosa and muscle to produce several possible effects. The actions of an individual fibre source depends to a large extent on its fermentability. The range of fermentability of different fibre is great and difficult to predict. Dietary fibre, however, can be roughly divided into those which are rapidly fermented, such as oligosaccharides, those which are more slowly fermented, such as gums, and those which are hardly fermented at all, such as wheat bran. The least fermentable fibres are the most likely to increase stool output. Dietary fibre which is highly fermentable is unlikely to have much effect on stool output but will affect bacterial fermentation products in the proximal colon and hence colonic and systemic physiology. Fibres which are slowly fermented may have a major influence in the distal colon even if they do not increase stool output significantly. Furthermore, the effect of each type of fibre is determined by dose.

Stool output

The dietary fibres which have the greatest effects on stool output are in general the least fermentable (90) These fibres probably act by virtue of their water holding capacity (WHC). The relationship between WHC and stool output is not simple. Dietary fibres with high WHC are those which are the most fermentable and are lost before they reach the rectum. There are exceptions such as ispaghula which has high WHC but resists fermentation. Moreover, one of the most reliable stool bulkers is wheat bran which has a WHC that is as low as the rest of faecal contents on a normal low fibre diet. It appears that the most important factor for a large effect on stool output is simply for the fibre to appear in stool. The effect is then dependent on the amount of fibre present as well as its residual WHC. The contribution of bacterial cells to faecal mass should not be forgotten, as the water content of bacteria is high. The effects of fibre are not restricted to increasing output. Dietary fibre has also a role in changing the consistency of the stool by increasing the water content and the plasticity, and increasing stool frequency.

Colonic motility and transit time

Certain fibres are known to have a laxative effect, in that their presence in the colon affects its motility and modifies colonic transit time. Two major mechanisms to explain this effect depend on the physicochemical properties and fermentative fate of fibre (91). These mechanisms refer to stimulation by the bulking effect of fibre as well as changes in the contractile activity and secretion of the colon (see Figure 6).

Increasing the volume of colonic contents distends the colon wall and stimulates propulsion of digesta through the activation of intramuscular mechanoreceptors. Dietary fibre can increase the faecal bulk by several mechanisms. First, the volume occupied by undegraded fibres adds to the volume of the rest of contents. This explains why the least fermentable fibres, such as wheat and corn bran, ispaghula or some algal polysaccharides, are particularly efficient laxatives. Also, these residues can trap water within their matrix, thus leading to a greater bulk. A third possible mechanism to increase intraluminal volume and stretch colonic muscle is the production of gases occurring during the fermentation of fibre.

Figure 6

Mechanisms of action of dietary fibre on colonic transit time

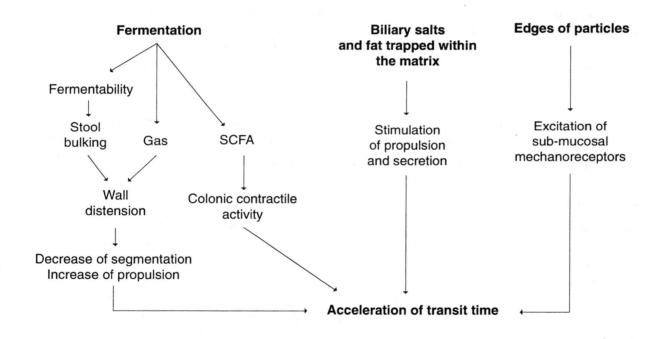

Source: Adapted from Salvador, V., Cherbut, C. (91)

In addition to their bulking effects, dietary fibre can reduce transit time by modulating contractile activity and water movements in the colon. Here again, they can act in several ways. First, the edges of solid particles can stimulate mechanoreceptors located in the submucosa and by that, modify the contractile pattern of the colon in favour of a greater propulsion of digesta, as has been shown with plastic particles. Fibre could also release compounds trapped in the small intestine (such as biliary salts or fatty acids) into the colon during fermentation. Such compounds have been shown to stimulate secretion and rectosigmoid motility.

Finally, a large part of fibre is fermented by microflora yielding several metabolites which can themselves influence colonic motility (92). For instance, SCFA stimulate contractions in the terminal ileum of humans and may also affect colonic motility as has been demonstrated with rats.

It has recently been appreciated that dietary starch bulks the stool (143,144,145), presumably because undigested starch provides energy for colonic bacterial growth. Thus, some of the faecal bulking effect of dietary fibre, at least in intact foods, could be due to the associated increase in starch delivery to the colon.

Vitamin and mineral absorption

Purified dietary fibres may reduce acutely the absorption of some vitamins and minerals by binding or entrapping them in the small intestinal lumen, however, there is little evidence that population groups consuming nutritionally adequate diets rich in high fibre foods, such as vegetarians, have any problems with vitamin or mineral deficiencies (170,171). Recent studies with calcium suggest that purified fibres reduce calcium availability in the small intestine, but that at least some of the calcium carried into the colon, bound to or entrapped by fibre, is released when the fibre is fermented (172) with the short chain fatty acid products of digestion facilitating calcium absorption from the distal colon and rectum (173).

CARBOHYDRATE FOOD INTAKE AND ENERGY BALANCE

Influence of carbohydrates on food intake

Food intake is regulated by the complex interaction of psychological and physiological events associated with ingestion. While the energy content of foods has an important role in determining the amount eaten, a number of other properties of foods also may be important. These include palatability, macronutrient composition, form of the food (solid vs liquid), how it is prepared, and its energy density (calories per gram).

Of key concern is whether the varying physiological responses to carbohydrates are associated with distinctive effects on food intake. Ways in which carbohydrates could influence intake include taste, chewing time, stomach distension, digestibility, absorption rate, hormonal changes, and metabolic signals arising as a result of carbohydrate utilization by different tissues. The roles of these various influences and the way that they interact to affect food intake are not well-understood.

It is useful to distinguish between "satiation" and "satiety." Satiation refers to the processes involved in the termination of a meal, whereas satiety refers to the effects of a food (often referred to as a preload) or a meal after eating has ended (93). Foods that are readily overeaten (i.e. have relatively little impact on satiation) are usually highly palatable and have high energy density. Most studies of carbohydrates have examined the effects on satiety, that is, how fixed amounts of carbohydrate or carbohydrate-rich foods impact subsequent food intake.

Sugars and food intake

The literature on the effects of sugars on the regulation of food intake has been recently reviewed (94). Some sugars are of particular interest because of the sweet taste they provide. While sweetness increases the palatability of foods, particularly when combined with fat, and therefore may increase the probability that sweet foods will be selected for consumption (95), there is no indication that sugar is associated with excessive food intake. Intake of sweet foods or drinks is limited by changes in the hedonic response to sweetness during consumption (96). Thus, to a hungry individual a sweet food will be rated as extremely pleasant in taste, but as consumption proceeds this rating of pleasantness declines. Ratings of foods with different tastes, for example, salty foods, will be unaffected by consumption of sweet foods. This "sensory-specific satiety" limits consumption of one type of food and helps to ensure that a variety of foods is consumed (97).

Many people believe that sugar and other carbohydrates contribute to overeating and obesity. Despite this popular belief, there is little direct evidence that obese individuals eat excessive quantities of sweet foods. Indeed, a number of studies show an inverse relationship between reported sugar consumption and degree of overweight (98). In a recent survey of the 10 favourite foods of a large sample of obese men and women, it was found that obese men listed mainly protein/fat sources (meat dishes) among their favourite foods, while obese women listed predominantly carbohydrate/fat sources (doughnuts, cookies, cake) and foods that are sweet. Preference for carbohydrates was not a standard feature of obesity. Rather preferences for major food sources of fat as opposed to carbohydrate may be a primary characteristic of human obesity syndromes (95,99). Thus, although there is little evidence that any of the various sugars are associated with obesity, sugars are often associated with a high-fat content in foods and serve to increase the palatability of fat, and fat is associated with obesity.

Starch and food intake

Variations in the starch in foods could affect the amount consumed or hunger and satiety. For example, the preparation method, the food source, and the amylose/amylopectin ratio can all lead to different glucose/insulin responses and hormonal profiles. Starchy foods vary widely in their glycemic response (the effect on blood glucose) from lente, a slow sustained glycemic response, to rapid increases in blood glucose (73). Slow digestion and absorption of carbohydrates helps to maintain steady blood glucose levels which can be beneficial to diabetics. High consumption of lente foods can also reduce serum triglycerides and improve lipid metabolism (100).

Altering the amylose/amylopectin ratio changes physiologic responses which could influence satiety. High-amylose starches are associated with a lower glycemic response than low-amylose starches, and they may also empty more slowly from the stomach. As would be predicted from these physiologic effects, increasing the amylose/amylopectin ratio has consistently been found to be associated with high satiety.

Predictions about how resistant starch would affect satiety are not straightforward. If similar amounts of resistant and regular starch are consumed, the resistant starch will deliver only about half the energy as the regular starch and one would expect decreased satiety and compensatory food intake. On the other hand, resistant starch may act like soluble fibre in that it could delay gastric emptying and prolong absorption which in turn could prolong satiety. When resistant starch (50g raw potato starch) was compared to an equal weight of pregelatinized potato starch consumed in a drink, the resistant starch was associated with a low glycemic response and was less satiating. Ratings of satiety and fullness returned to baseline fasting levels much more rapidly than they did with digestible starch (101).

Dietary fibre and food intake

There are a number of reasons why dietary fibre can reduce food intake: high-fibre foods take longer to eat; fibre decreases the energy density of food; some fibres such as guar gum and pectin slow gastric emptying; fibre may reduce the digestibility of food; there may be increased faecal loss of energy on high-fibre diets; and fibre may affect some gastrointestinal hormones that influence food intake (102).

The literature on this topic is complex because of the different types and doses of fibre that have been tested, and the wide variety of experimental protocols. This is illustrated by the previous discussion of the effects of resistant starch which is a type of dietary fibre. Nevertheless, there are a number of studies that show that high-fibre foods consumed either at breakfast or lunch significantly reduce intake at the next meal compared to low-fibre foods. A recent well-controlled study in which the effects of soluble or insoluble fibre supplementation at breakfast were compared, found that fibre supplementation (20g rather than 3g) was associated with a significant reduction in lunch intake. Total daily energy intake, however, was not affected by the quantity or type of fibre in the breakfast (103).

Energy and macronutrient balance

Maintaining a stable body weight requires achieving energy balance, where the amount of energy ingested equals the amount of energy expended. While obesity can only develop when energy intake exceeds energy expenditure (104), efforts to attribute obesity solely to a high level of energy intake or to a low level of energy expenditure have been unsuccessful. Obesity could develop slowly from a small, sustained positive energy balance produced by some combination of increased energy intake and decreased physical activity or could result from periodic bouts of positive energy balance achieved by temporary increases in intake or decreases in physical activity.

Achieving body weight regulation requires more than achieving energy balance; it also requires that macronutrient balance be achieved. Macronutrient balance means that the intake of each macronutrient is equal to its oxidation. If this is not the case for a particular macronutrient, body stores of that macronutrient will change. For a weight-stable individual this means that the composition of fuel oxidized is equal to the composition of energy ingested. When the state of energy and macronutrient balance is disrupted (e.g. overfeeding, altering chronic level of physical activity), the body attempts to restore this state of homeostasis. In such cases, the differences in the rapidity with which balance of each macronutrient is restored has important implications for the role of diet composition in body weight regulation.

The hierarchy for substrate oxidation

The fuel for energy expenditure is supplied by protein, carbohydrate and fat. This fuel can be supplied by the diet or can come from body energy stores. There appears to be a hierarchy for substrate oxidation which is determined by the storage capability of the body for each macronutrient, the energy costs of converting a macronutrient to a form with greater storage capacity, and by specific fuel needs of certain tissues. Alcohol has highest priority for oxidation because there is no body storage pool and conversion of alcohol to fat is energetically expensive. Amino acids are next in the oxidative hierarchy. Again, there is not a specific storage pool for amino acids. Body proteins are functional in nature and do not serve as a storage depot for amino acids. Carbohydrates are third in the oxidative hierarchy. There is a limited capacity to store carbohydrate as glycogen (a typical adult male can store approximately 500 g of glycogen, predominantly in muscle and liver) and conversion of carbohydrate to fat is energetically expensive. Carbohydrate is also somewhat unique in that it is an obligatory fuel for the central nervous system and the formed blood elements (e.g. red blood cells). In contrast to the other macronutrients there a virtually unlimited storage capacity for fat (largely in adipose tissue). The efficiency of storage of dietary fat in adipose tissue is very high (96-98%). Unlike carbohydrate, fat is not a unique fuel source for any body tissue.

Because of their oxidative priority, the body has an exceptional ability to maintain alcohol and protein balance across a wide range of intake of each. Because carbohydrate stores represent a small proportion of daily carbohydrate intake and because net *de novo* lipogenesis from carbohydrate does not occur to an appreciable extent under normal circumstances (105,106), carbohydrate oxidation closely matches carbohydrate intake. Carbohydrate balance appears to be well maintained across a wide range of carbohydrate intake. Unlike other macronutrients, fat does not promote its own oxidation and the amount of fat which is oxidized is the difference between total energy needs and oxidation of the other priority fuels.

Obesity and nutrient balance

The body's ability to maintain energy and nutrient balance is dependent upon a complex regulatory system that allows the body to achieve and maintain a steady-state of energy and nutrient balance. Sustained increases in energy intake can lead to increased body weight and an accompanying increase in energy expenditure. Body weight will stabilize and energy balance will be achieved when energy expenditure is increased to the level of energy intake. Conversely, a decrease in energy intake will disrupt energy balance and produce a loss of body weight accompanied by a reduction in energy expenditure. Body weight will stabilize when energy expenditure declines to the level of energy intake.

It may be more useful in understanding body weight regulation to examine how the body achieves macronutrient balance. As discussed earlier, acute changes in intake of alcohol, protein, or carbohydrate are rapidly balanced by changes in oxidation of each. In contrast, fat oxidation is not tightly linked to fat intake. As a consequence, positive or negative energy balance are largely conditions of positive or negative fat balance. Thus, the point at which a stable body weight and body composition is reached and defended is that point at which fat balance is achieved.

The two major factors which influence fat balance are amount and composition of food eaten and the total amount of physical activity. Positive fat balance can be produced by overconsumption of energy or restriction of physical activity. Positive fat balance will occur when any type of diet is overconsumed. During carbohydrate overfeeding, for example, carbohydrate oxidation increases to maintain carbohydrate balance, but because carbohydrate is providing more fuel for oxidative needs, fat oxidation is providing less than usual, creating positive fat balance (107).

Negative fat balance can result from underconsumption of total energy or fat or by an increase in the level of physical activity. During underconsumption of energy, the supply of the priority metabolic fuels (carbohydrate and protein) are insufficient to meet the body's energy needs. Thus, the remaining energy needs are met by fat oxidation which comes largely from endogenous fat stores. An increase in the level of physical activity will increase total energy requirements with the additional energy needs being met by increased fat oxidation.

Fat balance and body weight stability

There are two mechanisms by which a new steady-state of body weight and body composition achieved following a positive or negative perturbation in fat balance. First, changes in behaviour can lead to adjustments in either intake or oxidation of fat (e.g. altering total energy or fat intake and altering physical activity). Second, in the absence of sufficient behaviour changes, fat oxidation will be altered following alterations in the body fat mass. As an example of behavioural adjustments, the negative fat balance produced by reducing energy intake could be eliminated totally by a compensatory reduction in physical activity. As an example of metabolic adjustments, overconsumption of total energy and fat will produce positive energy balance. If behavioural adjustments are absent or insufficient, increases in the body fat mass will result. Increased body fat mass is associated with increased levels of circulating free fatty acids which elevate total fat oxidation. Thus, a stable body weight will be reached at the point where the body fat mass has increased sufficiently so that fat oxidation equals fat intake.

Metabolic differences between carbohydrate and fat

Based on known differences in macronutrient metabolism, we can begin to predict how the composition of the diet, and specifically the carbohydrate to fat ratio of the diet, might impact upon body weight regulation. It must be realized that the pathways by which nutrients are metabolized (particularly carbohydrate) vary with the overall state of energy balance and this must be considered when predicting the impact of diet composition. For example, conversion of carbohydrate to fat would occur during situations of excess carbohydrate intake and not under situations of normal or below normal intake.

Changing diet composition with no energy intake change

Altering diet composition without a change in total energy intake should have relatively modest effects on body weight and body fat content. There are at least two ways that such a change in diet composition could affect body weight. First, the thermic effect of carbohydrate is greater than the thermic effect of fat. Changing to a lower fat diet (assuming total energy and protein intake remain constant) means changing to a higher carbohydrate diet, which will increase total energy expenditure. The magnitude of increase in energy expenditure depends on the magnitude of change of the carbohydrate/fat ratio, but is probably relatively small and of questionable importance in body weight regulation for reducing dietary fat from 35-40% to 20-25% of total energy intake. Second, altering the carbohydrate/fat ratio of the diet requires that substrate oxidation rates be readjusted to the new macronutrient intakes. If total energy expenditure is not changed, these changes occur relatively rapidly, with carbohydrate and protein balance being reachieved more quickly than fat balance (108,109). Negative fat balance and some loss of body fat will occur until fat balance is reachieved. It is difficult to predict the rapidity with which fat balance will be reachieved following a reduction in fat (and an accompanying increase in carbohydrate intake).

Effects of diet composition during positive energy balance

It is during periods of positive energy balance that differences in carbohydrate and fat have the greatest impact upon body weight regulation. This is because of differences in the efficiency of metabolic pathways involved in disposing of excess carbohydrate vs fat. One study (107) demonstrated that while the majority of excess energy is stored regardless of its composition, a greater proportion of excess energy is stored when the excess is from fat as compared to when the excess is from carbohydrate. This is a clear example of a situation where fat intake leads to more body energy storage than the same amount of energy from carbohydrate.

Total energy expenditure increases more with carbohydrate overfeeding than with fat overfeeding. This is because carbohydrate oxidation increases to a greater extent than fat oxidation decreases during carbohydrate overfeeding. The difference between carbohydrate and fat in the proportion of excess energy stored is greatest during the first week of overfeeding. This suggests that the more sustained the overfeeding, the less the difference between carbohydrate and fat overfeeding. If obesity develops due to brief, periodic episodes of overeating, differences between fat and carbohydrate are likely to be more important than if obesity develops from sustained positive energy balance.

Carbohydrate type and body weight regulation

The effects of different types of carbohydrates on body weight regulation have been reviewed recently (110). While there are clear differences in metabolism of carbohydrates and fat that could affect body weight regulation, there do not appear to be such metabolic differences between types of carbohydrate. The majority of comparisons have been made between simple sugars and complex carbohydrates. There is little scientific support for the commonly held perception that consumption of high amounts of simple sugar contributes to obesity. There is no evidence that simple sugars are used with a different efficiency than complex carbohydrates (other than dietary fibre or resistant oligosaccharides). While there is substantial data suggesting that high levels of dietary fat intake are associated with high levels of obesity, at present there is no reason to believe that high intake of simple sugar is associated with high levels of obesity.

Does carbohydrate make you fat?

The idea that increased insulin concentrations subsequent to carbohydrate intake lead to conversion of significant amounts of carbohydrate to fat is misleading. First, it takes an extreme excess of carbohydrate to produce *de novo* lipogenesis, and even under these conditions, very little net fat is produced from carbohydrate. Second, the idea that persons with insulin resistance are particularly prone to become obese when eating high carbohydrate diets is unsubstantiated by scientific evidence. In fact, low-fat, high-carbohydrate diets are commonly recommended to prevent further weight gain for these individuals who are at risk to develop non-insulin dependent diabetes and coronary heart disease. Finally, substantial data suggest that voluntary energy intake is higher in many people when the diet is high in fat content and low in carbohydrate content. Excess consumption of energy in any form leads to accumulation of body fat. There is no serious scientific evidence to suggest, however, that diets high in carbohydrate promote weight gain when consumed in amounts which do not exceed energy requirements.

Prevention of obesity

Because excess dietary fat is stored more efficiently than excess dietary carbohydrate, eating a low fat diet may be helpful in obesity prevention. If one assumes that everyone overeats occasionally, less of the excess energy will be stored as adipose tissue if a low fat diet is consumed than a high fat diet. It remains prudent to recommend a high carbohydrate diet for body weight maintenance. Diets high in fat are likely to promote excess energy consumption and excess dietary fat is stored as adipose tissue with extremely high efficiency. Eating a high carbohydrate diet reduces the likelihood of overeating and, if overeating occurs, results in slightly less of the excess energy being stored as adipose tissue.

Alternative sweeteners

Dietary carbohydrates responsible for sweet taste are often replaced or substituted to varying extents by alternative sweeteners. The main reasons are to reduce the energy content of the diet, to minimise postprandial blood glucose fluctuations, to reduce cariogenicity, and to reduce cost.

Alternative sweeteners are defined as sweeteners other than sucrose. The term *sweetener* is mostly used for the high-intensity sweeteners (174) or for "any substance other than a carbohydrate whose primary sensory characteristic is sweet"(175), but sometimes to also collectively describe nutritive and non-nutritive sweeteners. The nutritive sweeteners are the mono- and disaccharide sugars and a large variety of carbohydrate sweeteners that occur naturally in foods or are added in purified form (174).

The two main groups of alternative sweeteners that are used as sucrose substitutes or replacers, and classified on the basis of their function in foods, are the high intensity "non-nutritive" sweeteners and the "nutritive" bulk sweeteners or "sugar bulking" agents.

Non-nutritive sweeteners

Alternative sweeteners which are non-nutritive, non-carbohydrate, very low in calories and with an intense sweet taste, have been further grouped into three classes (176). First, the naturally occurring compounds such as monellin, thaumatin, miraculin, stevioside, steviol, etc., of which more than 30 have been identified and described. The second group includes the synthetic compounds saccharin, cyclamate, acesulfame, and others. The third group has two semi-synthetic compounds, neohesperidin dihydrochalcone (NHDC) and the dipeptide aspartylphenylalanine, also known as aspartame.

Nutritive sweeteners

Other alternative sweeteners are low-energy, bulk, sugar (sucrose) substitutes which are used not only for their sweet taste, but also to replace intrinsic functions of sugar in baked products, ice cream, frozen desserts, and other processed foods. These sugar substitutes are carbohydrates and are usually classified as nutritive sweeteners. They include glucose (dextrose), liquid glucose, high fructose syrups, liquid fructose, crystalline fructose, corn syrup, corn syrup solids, concentrated grape juice, invert sugar, invert syrups (174,175), and polyols, which are polyhydric alcohols produced by the hydrogenation of the corresponding reducing sugars.

THE ROLE OF CARBOHYDRATES IN EXERCISE AND PHYSICAL PERFORMANCE

Introduction

Interest in the influences of food on the capacity for physical activity is as old as mankind. From earliest times, certain foods were regarded as essential preparation for strenuous physical activity. In a recent consensus conference on food, nutrition and sports performance, carbohydrate containing foods were identified as having the most significant impact on exercise performance. The nutritional importance of protein, as a fuel for exercise and as a contributor to strength development, has been over emphasized, whereas the fluid intake has been, by comparison, underplayed (183).

Most studies on the influence of carbohydrate intake on exercise performance have been conducted in laboratories using either cycling or treadmill running. Performance is usually assessed as either the time to exhaustion (endurance capacity) during exercise of constant intensity, or the time to run a predetermined distance or complete a prescribed workload (performance) in the shortest time possible. In some studies, the investigators have combined the elements of both endurance capacity and performance in one protocol in order to try to simulate an activity pattern common in sports. For example, running at a constant submaximal pace for an hour or more and then completing a set distance in as fast a time as possible; or cycling at a constant submaximal workload and after an hour pedalling as fast as possible to complete a set work load as quickly as possible. The division between endurance capacity and endurance performance is artificial because in any real life endurance race or event, both endurance capacity and pace are required in order to be successful. Nevertheless, by obtaining a better understanding of simple endurance capacity, we can get a clearer picture of the essential determinants of endurance performance.

Some general dietary considerations

Health professionals argue that a healthy diet is one which provides us with at least 50% of our daily energy intake in the form of carbohydrates, 35 % or less from fats and the remainder from proteins. The common message is that we should move from high fat meat-based diets to those that are made up of more carbohydrates and fresh fruits and vegetables. The consensus view on the diet for athletes and active people is that it should include more carbohydrate-containing foods than recommended by the health professionals. Their diets should be such that about 60% of their daily energy intake is obtained from carbohydrates, 30 % or less from fat and 10 to 15 % from proteins (183).

Carbohydrate diets and endurance capacity

An early study exploring the link between diet and exercise capacity found that after a period on a high carbohydrate diet, endurance capacity on a cycle ergometer, doubled in comparison with the exercise times achieved after consuming a normal mixed diet. In contrast, a fat and protein diet reduced exercise capacity to almost half that achieved after normal mixed diets. This clearly showed the benefits of eating a high-carbohydrate diet before prolonged exercise and was the first to establish importance of the carbohydrate content in the diets of athletes preparing for competition.

The benefits of carbohydrate loading before prolonged submaximal exercise have been shown mainly during cycling. A link was demonstrated between endurance performance during cycle ergometry and pre-exercise muscle glycogen concentration (184). The importance of muscle glycogen during prolonged exercise was confirmed in subsequent studies which showed that fatigue occurs when muscle glycogen concentrations are reduced to low values (185-187). Therefore, it is not surprising that attempts were made to find methods of increasing muscle glycogen stores in preparation for prolonged exercise. One study (188) examined the influence of different nutritional states on the resynthesis of glycogen during recovery from prolonged exhaustive exercise. It found that a diet low in carbohydrate, and high in fat and protein for 2 to 3 days after prolonged submaximal exercise, produced a delayed muscle glycogen resynthesis, but when this was followed by a high carbohydrate diet for the same period of time, glycogen supercompensation occurred (see Figure 7). This dietary manipulation not only increased the pre-exercise muscle glycogen concentration but also resulted in a significant improvement in endurance capacity (see Figure 8). Although this original method of carbohydrate-loading was recommended as part of the preparation for endurance competitions, the low carbohydrate, high fat and protein phase of the diet is an unpleasant experience. Therefore, alternative ways were explored to increase the pre-exercise glycogen stores without including a period on a diet high in fat and protein (189). It was found that a carbohydrate-rich diet consumed for 3 days prior to competition, accompanied by a decrease in training intensity, resulted in increased muscle glycogen concentrations of the same magnitude as those achieved with the traditional carbohydrate loading procedure.

Figure 7

**Muscle glycogen concentrations before
and after constant load cycling to exhaustion,
following three dietary conditions**

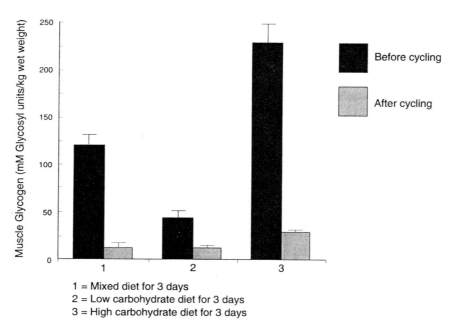

Source: Adapted from Bergstrom, J., Hermansen, L., Hultman, E., Saltin, B. (188)

There have been fewer studies on the influence of carbohydrate loading and endurance capacity during running. In one of the few running studies, the question of what type of carbohydrate should be consumed in preparation for prolonged exercise was considered (190). The runners' normal mixed diets were modified by providing either additional protein, complex carbohydrates or simple carbohydrates. The 'complex' carbohydrate group supplemented their normal mixed diet with bread, potatoes, rice or pasta. The 'simple' carbohydrate group ate their normal mixed diet but increased their carbohydrate intake with chocolates. Running times increased after both high carbohydrate diets. The complex carbohydrate group improved their running times by 26%, and the simple carbohydrate group improved by 23%. There was no improvement in the performance times of the protein group, confirming that the carbohydrate content of the diet is the important nutrient and that the changes were not simply the consequence of a greater energy intake.

Figure 8

Cycling time to exhaustion at constant load under three dietary conditions

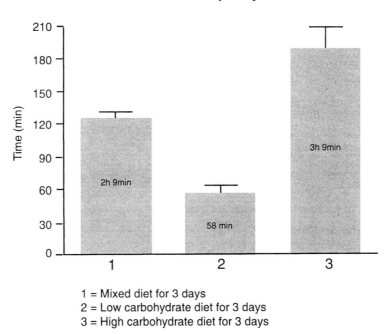

Diet and Endurance Capacity

1 = Mixed diet for 3 days
2 = Low carbohydrate diet for 3 days
3 = High carbohydrate diet for 3 days

Source: Adapted from Bergstrom, J., Hermansen, L., Hultman, E., Saltin, B. (188)

Carbohydrate diets and endurance performance

In a recent study, the influence of carbohydrate loading on running performance during a simulated 30-km race was conducted using a laboratory treadmill (191). One of the aims of this study was to determine at what point during the race runners began to show signs of fatigue and how this was modified by dietary manipulation. The treadmill was instrumented so that the subjects controlled their own speeds using a light-weight hand-held switch.

Changes in speed, time, and distance elapsed were all displayed on a computer screen in full view of the subjects. The runners were divided into two groups after the first 30-km treadmill time trial. One group increased their carbohydrate intake during the 7 day recovery period, whereas the other group ate additional protein and fat in order to match the increased energy intakes of the carbohydrate group. Although there was no overall improvement in performance times for the two groups, the carbohydrate group ran faster during the last 10 km of the simulated race. Furthermore, eight of the nine runners in the carbohydrate group had faster times for 30 km than during their first attempt, and better times than the control group. Even though the carbohydrate group ran faster than the control group, after carbohydrate loading they had lower adrenaline concentrations. This was attributed to the carbohydrate loading and subsequent maintenance of normal blood glucose concentrations throughout the race. Noradrenaline concentrations increased, as expected, during the simulated 30-km races following normal dietary conditions and after carbohydrate loading.

Carbohydrate diets and high intensity exercise

More people participate, at a recreational level, in 'multiple-sprint' sports (such as soccer, hockey, tennis, basketball and rugby), than endurance (cycling, swimming or running). These multiple-sprint sports involve a mixture of brief periods of exercise of maximum intensity followed by recovery periods of rest or light activity, and last up to 90 minutes. Only a limited amount of information is available, however, on the influence of diet on exercise of maximal intensity and brief duration. One of the reasons for the limited amount of research on this topic has been the lack of suitable laboratory methods for studying the metabolic and physiological responses to maximal exercise. Inexpensive micro-computers are now widely available, and so they are used to record rapid changes in power outputs during maximal exercise of short duration.

Even though there is rapid utilization of muscle glycogen during several brief periods of maximal exercise, the rate of glycogenolysis decreases as exercise continues. For example, in a series of 10 maximal sprints of 6-second duration and 30-second recovery on a cycle ergometer, glycogen degradation was reduced by half during the last sprint (192). This glycogen sparing is probably the consequence of an increase in the aerobic metabolism of glycogen and free fatty acids (193).

Performance during sports which involve several brief sprints may not be improved by carbohydrate loading. Sports which demand that their participants perform a combination of submaximal running and brief periods of sprinting, such as soccer, reduces muscle glycogen concentrations to critically low values. Performance is impaired when this occurs, and so carbohydrate loading would probably be of benefit to participants in multiple-sprint sports (194).

Composition of pre-exercise meals

The type of the carbohydrate in pre-exercise meals and their influences on subsequent endurance capacity has, until recently, received too little attention. The description of carbohydrates as either simple or complex is an inadequate way of classifying them. A metabolically more informative way of describing carbohydrates is the degree to which they raise blood glucose concentrations. Carbohydrates which produce a large increase in blood glucose concentration, in response to a standard amount of carbohydrate (50g), are classified as having a high glycemic index. The metabolic response during exercise is different as a consequence of the glycemic indices of the carbohydrates consumed preceding the exercise (195), and so the choice of carbohydrate in pre-competition meals could have an effect on performance.

In one study on the influence of high and low glycemic index carbohydrate foods on exercise capacity, the low glycemic index carbohydrate appeared to improve endurance capacity to a greater extent than the high glycemic index food (196). This study used lentils as the low glycemic index food, with potatoes and glucose as the high glycemic index foods, and compared the responses to these after drinking a glucose solution or plain water.

Eating a high fat meal three to four hours before exercise is not recommended as a nutritional preparation for endurance competitions because these meals take a longer time to digest. There is some evidence from animal studies to suggest that increased fat intake will result in a lower than normal oxidation of carbohydrate during exercise. If this glycogen sparing did occur following a high fat meal then it would be expected to delay the onset of fatigue in a similar manner to consuming carbohydrate-rich meals before exercise. A recent study has attempted to answer this question by comparing the endurance performances of subjects following isocaloric high fat or high carbohydrate meals, four hours before submaximal exercise (197). The pre-exercise meals contained approximately 280g of carbohydrate in the high carbohydrate meal and 84g in the high fat meal. There was no statistically significant difference between the endurance times from the high carbohydrate and high fat (low carbohydrate) meals (197).

Recovery from exercise

Recovery from exercise is not a passive process. Tissues undergo repair and reproduction, fluid balance is restored and substrate stores are replaced. Carbohydrate replacement is one of the most important events during recovery. When several days separate periods of exercise or participation in sport, a normal mixed diet containing about 4 to 5 g/kg body weight (BW) of carbohydrate is sufficient to replace muscle glycogen stores. However, daily training or competition makes considerable demands on the body's carbohydrate stores. Therefore, the normally high carbohydrate intake of athletes may not be enough to prevent a gradual reduction in this important fuel store. For example, even when the daily carbohydrate intake is 5 g/kg BW, cycling or running for an hour each day gradually delays the daily restoration of muscle glycogen stores (198). Increasing the carbohydrate intake to 8 g/kg BW per day may not be enough to prevent a significant reduction in muscle glycogen concentrations after 5 successive days of hard training (199). These studies underline the importance of prescribing adequate amounts of carbohydrate for athletes in training and justifies the need for more frequent recovery days between periods of intense training.

Summary

The clear message from over a half a century of research on the links between food, nutrition and exercise capacity is that next to natural talent and appropriate training, a high carbohydrate diet and adequate fluid intake to avoid dehydration are the two most important elements in the formula for successful participation in sport. Of course, there is an underlying assumption that athletes normally eat a well-balanced diet made up of a wide variety of foods, and contains sufficient energy to cover their needs.

SUGAR AND HUMAN BEHAVIOUR

Introduction

The assertion that foods containing sugar might have an adverse effect on behaviour was first raised in 1922 by Shannon (200). This concept was further elaborated in 1947 by Randolph (201) in his description of the tension fatigue syndrome. Sugar later appeared in the 1970's as a major offending agent when the lay literature provided considerable coverage to the condition called functional reactive hypoglycemia (202). In establishing sugar as a major dietary component, it is important to review if a relationship does exist between sugar and behaviour. The first and most prominently believed relationship is that between sucrose and hyperactivity and/or aggressive behaviours. A second less well-known relationship has been suggested between glucose and enhanced memory, particularly in elderly individuals. A third reported relationship has been sugar's effect on the opposite of hyperactivity, namely sedation.

Sugar and hyperactivity

The belief in the relationship between sugar and hyperactivity is based on two theories. The first, that hyperactivity is a possible allergic response to refined sugar, was conceived of in the first half of this century as the tension-fatigue syndrome, a behavioural correlate to the vomiting reaction to milk proteins (203). The second suggested etiology is that some children may experience functional reactive hypoglycemia similar to that seen in adults (204). Individuals with functional reactive hypoglycemia experience glucose levels in the hypoglycemic range while on diets high in carbohydrates. Consuming diets high in proteins seems to prevent this condition. It was theorized that children would display increased motor activity at low blood glucose levels.

Most intervention research has entailed controlled double-blinded challenge studies. Children receive challenges with foods or drinks containing sucrose or an artificial sweetener where the children, their parents and the researchers are not aware of the composition of the foods or drink and their behaviour and cognitive performance is closely assessed within the few hours after ingestion. In reviewing these studies, there are some important considerations.

The first consideration in any rigorous study is the characteristics of the subject. In examining the effects of sugar, the subjects have been children with a wide array of characteristics. Studies have involved normal children, children historically identified as behaving poorly after sugar ingestion, children diagnosed with hyperactivity or attention deficit disorders, and aggressive or delinquent children. The studies have used subjects ranging in age from preschoolers to adolescents.

The second consideration is the type or quantity of sugar likely to affect behaviour. For this there are few, if any, guidelines. Sucrose has been the most prominent sweetening agent used although many foods are now sweetened with corn sweeteners, i.e. fructose. Fructose and glucose have been included in a few of the studies. Most challenge studies have employed the quantity used in glucose tolerance tests (1.75 gm/kg) although doses as high as 5.6 gm/kg have been studied.

The diet condition prior to challenge is a third consideration. This issue, has been a concern, particularly regarding the specific manipulation of the carbohydrate to protein or fat ratio. There has, however, been a great deal of variation among studies, ranging from no diet control to restricted diets. It is expected, however, that with the degree of variation present in the studies, it would be possible to detect responses if pre-existing diets were a factor.

The final important issue is the measurement of the proposed effects of refined sugar. Most measures have focused on the behaviour of children with attention deficit hyperactivity disorder who are characterized as having a short attention span, impulsive behaviour and increased motor activity compared to other children. The studies have utilized parent and/or teacher report to assess behaviour. Numerous behaviour rating scales with reasonable psychometric properties were used depending on age and range of behaviours. Other neuropsychological measures have also been employed to assess vigilance, impulsivity, memory and motor skills. Some studies have employed electronic motion detector devices to record activity level. There have also been direct observations and recordings of behaviours for short segments of time by independent observers and rating scales completed by independent observers. These have been important because, while parents are good reporters of their children's behaviours and have been blinded to conditions, they are not independent and do affect their children's behaviours.

A meta-analysis of 23 studies which had been conducted over a period of 12 years from 1982 to 1994 has been completed (205), to test the hypothesis that sugar (mainly sucrose) affects the behaviour or cognitive performance of children. This analysis did not find support for the hypothesis. In conclusion, there is little objective evidence to suggest that sugar significantly alters the behaviour or cognitive performance of children. It is not appropriate to recommend restricting a child's sugar intake for the purpose of trying to control their behaviour. If behaviour problems exist, it is important to identify the underlying reasons and to seek the existing and more rigorously established interventions for their treatment.

Glucose and memory

There is increasing evidence that sugar, glucose specifically, can influence central nervous system activity. Although memory enhancement was not demonstrated in any of the challenge studies which measured memory in children, there is evidence that glucose levels influence memory functioning in rats and humans, locomotor activity and sleep patterns in rats, and the distress associated with painful procedures in human infants. The focus of research in this area has been to establish how glucose acts to mediate these effects.

Since the retention of memory is an important central nervous system function in the process of cognition, central nervous system mechanisms salient to this function such as noradrenergic and cholinergic systems have been investigated. To investigate the positive effects of epinephrine on memory processing, one study systematically examined the effects of glucose on both animal and human subjects. The study (206) employed a foot shock avoidance task on rats, and observed, similar to the epinephrine effects, significantly improved retention in animals who received 10 to 100 mg/kg injection of glucose immediately after training. No effect was observed if the injection was delayed by one hour or if higher or lower doses were used. In a subsequent study (207), glucose was shown to have similar effects to other memory modulators in that its administration with low foot shock training enhanced the rats' memory storage while its administration with high foot shock training impaired retention possibly due to endogenous levels of epinephrine produced by the foot shock.

Extending the postulate that glucose improves memory functioning to a human population, one study (208) demonstrated significantly improved memory processing via a standardized measure in nine of eleven elderly human subjects after administration of oral glucose versus placebo. Further, a study found that enhancement of memory in elderly humans twenty-four hours after learning was significantly improved by glucose administration before or after the learning task (209). This may be similar to the finding in rats where memory potentiation in elderly rats was more marked than that demonstrated in a young adult rat population (210). None of the studies of sugar in children showed any effect on memory while those completed with elderly subjects did. However, it is important to note that most of the child studies used sucrose and only a few of them specifically tested memory.

In summary, there is evidence that glucose is discretely involved in neuroendocrine modulation of memory storage in both rats and humans. This influence is best demonstrated in elderly subjects. Further, one site of action of glucose is the medial septum which is rich with communications to the hippocampus. Although, the precise mechanism of the effects of glucose on memory are not yet established, these findings may have far reaching implications for pharmacologic treatment of memory impairments resulting from old age or head trauma. As of now the clinical implications of these findings have yet to be defined. Much more extensive research is required before any conclusions about clinically relevant implications can be drawn.

Summary

It appears clear that there is little evidence to support the claim that refined sugar intake has a significant influence on the behaviour or cognitive performance in children as popularly supposed. There may be a few children with idiosyncratic reactions or rare allergic syndromes who may respond adversely, but this has yet to be substantiated by carefully controlled research. The relationship of glucose to the improvement of memory processing appears clear. Further research is required to define its clinical relevance and to elucidate the mechanisms involved.

CARBOHYDRATES AND NON-COMMUNICABLE DISEASES .

Carbohydrates and diabetes

The role of dietary factors in the aetiology of non-insulin dependent diabetes (NIDDM) has been the subject of many epidemiological studies. It is important to emphasize that there are major difficulties in assessing nutritional aetiologies of any chronic disease. In addition to the problems inherent in various epidemiological approaches (ecological studies, case control and cohort studies), the instruments for measuring intake of food and nutrients (diet records, 24-hour recalls and food frequency questionnaires) all have limitations. Feeding studies in animals and humans may help to confirm or refute observations made in epidemiological studies.

Carbohydrates and dietary fibre in the aetiology of diabetes

The suggestion that refined carbohydrates, and sugars in particular, might be involved in the aetiology of NIDDM dates back to the writings of early Indian physicians. Over 40 studies have examined the role of sugars in the aetiology of NIDDM, with about half suggesting a positive association and a comparable number suggesting no association. Some have even suggested an inverse association between diabetes incidence and sucrose intake (111). Further evidence to suggest that sucrose is not an important contributing factor in the aetiology of NIDDM comes from carefully controlled studies in people with NIDDM (112). Isoenergetic substitution of moderate amounts of sucrose in the diets of individuals participating in randomized cross-over experiments do not result in deterioration in glycemic control. There is similarly little evidence that readily digested starchy foods increase the risk of developing NIDDM.

On the other hand, there is rather more support for the suggestion that foods rich in slowly digested or resistant starch or high in soluble dietary fibre might be protective. Countries with high intakes of these foods have low rates of diabetes and Trowell drew attention to the fact that the reduced mortality rates for diabetes during and after the Second World War parallelled the increased intake of dietary fibre during that period (113). These observations on their own provide no more evidence for a protective role for these foods than do comparable studies suggesting a causal role of sucrose. However, there is some corroborative evidence for a protective role of dietary fibre (non-starch polysaccharide) and slowly absorbed or resistant starch and the foods which are rich in these nutrients.

One study has shown that consumption of legumes rich in soluble dietary fibre was inversely associated with risk of glucose intolerance (114). Experimental studies provide further confirmation. In controlled experiments, diets high in soluble fibre-rich foods (115) or foods with a low glycemic index are associated with improved diurnal blood glucose profiles as well as long term overall improvement in glycemic control as evidenced by reduced levels of glycated haemoglobin (116). Some other studies provide indirect support for this hypothesis. Diabetes risk appears to be lower in vegetarians than in those who are not vegetarians (117). The diet of vegetarians is characterised by a high intake of dietary fibre, but differs in other ways from that of non-vegetarians. In addition to not eating meat and animal products, vegetarians also have less saturated fat, more polyunsaturated fat and a diet which differs in micronutrient composition when compared with non-vegetarians.

Not all studies have been able to confirm the protective effect of dietary fibre. For example, in two studies, no associations were found between intakes of carbohydrate or fibre and the risk of diabetes. Despite these negative findings (118) the overall weight of evidence suggests that individuals who consume diets rich in soluble dietary fibre or which have a low glycemic index are likely to be at reduced risk of developing diabetes. Conclusive evidence of a causal association is unlikely to be forthcoming.

Carbohydrates in the treatment of diabetes

Diabetic dietary recommendations - general principles

Before the discovery of insulin in the 1920s, radical restriction of dietary carbohydrate was the cornerstone of diabetes treatment. However, even after widespread availability of insulin, people with insulin-dependent diabetes mellitus (IDDM) were recommended to consume diets in which carbohydrate provided less that 40% total energy. It is difficult to establish the reason for this advice since there is no experimental data proving the benefits of carbohydrate restriction for people who are adequately insulinised. Carbohydrate restriction will lead to improvement in glycemic control in overweight NIDDM patients if such restriction is accompanied by weight loss but these observations provide no scientific justification for the value of restricting carbohydrate-containing foods. Dietary recommendations for the management of diabetes have been made in most countries, but those of the American Diabetes Association and European Association for the Study of Diabetes have been particularly widely quoted (119,120). The two sets of recommendations are in broad agreement. (See Table 10 for carbohydrate dietary recommendations for diabetes).

Carbohydrate and dietary fibre intake for diabetes

In the 1970s a series of studies from various research groups showed that a high carbohydrate diet (up to 60% total energy from carbohydrate) was associated with improved glycemic control and reduced levels of LDL cholesterol when compared with a low carbohydrate diet (40% total energy). These findings, together with the observation that people with diabetes in societies which traditionally consume a high carbohydrate diet have low rates of ischaemic heart disease (IHD), led some official diabetes organizations to recommend a change from the traditional low carbohydrate to a high carbohydrate diet.

Sugars

Avoidance of 'simple sugars', especially sucrose has undoubtedly been the most widely recommended component of the diabetic dietary recommendations. This is based on the incorrect assumption, however, that sugars will aggravate hyperglycemia to a greater extent than other carbohydrates. Indeed there is evidence to the contrary. It has long been known that blood glucose levels following a sucrose or fructose load are lower than after a comparable oral glucose load or starchy foods containing a similar amount of carbohydrate (121). This observation led to longer term studies in which diets including sucrose within mixed meals were compared with sucrose-free diets. The result of such studies confirmed that moderate intakes of sucrose (up to about 50g daily) can be incorporated into the diets of people with diabetes provided the sucrose is consumed as part of a meal and does not displace fibre-rich carbohydrate (112). These findings apply to those with both insulin-dependent and non-insulin-dependent diabetes.

TABLE 10
Some dietary recommendations for diabetes

Components of dietary energy	- Saturated fatty acids, <10% of total energy - ω-6 polyunsaturated fatty acids, <10% of total energy - Protein, 10-20% of total energy - Carbohydrate and cis-monounsaturated fatty acids, for the remainder
Carbohydrate issues	- Low glycemic index foods and those rich in soluble fibre recommended - Vegetables, fruits, pulses and cereal-derived foods preferred - Sucrose, <10% total energy acceptable in certain circumstances - Timing of intake essential for those on insulin
Special 'diabetic' and 'dietetic' foods	- Non-alcoholic beverages sweetened with non-nutritive sweeteners are useful - Other special foods not encouraged - No particular need of fructose and other 'special' nutritive sweeteners over sucrose

General advice regarding carbohydrate intake

While some foods have predictable and consistent glycemic indices, others will vary from country to country or indeed sometimes widely within a single country. Locally determined information is therefore essential. However, with regard to carbohydrate-containing foods one may in summary say that the staple cereals, breads, pasta, pulses, vegetables and fruit are generally appropriate sources of carbohydrate for people with diabetes. Such foods should form a major component of all meals and snacks. They should not adversely influence blood glucose levels in the short term, and may help to achieve optimum glycemic control in the long term. In addition, they are usually good sources of a wide range of essential macronutrients. Fibre-depleted starchy foods, foods rich in simple sugars, sucrose and other added sugars need not necessarily be totally excluded but should generally be restricted.

Carbohydrates and cardiovascular disease

History and epidemiology of carbohydrates and cardiovascular disease (CVD)

The hunter-gatherer diet had in excess of 50% of its energy from carbohydrate (122) and cardiovascular disease as we know it today, with underlying atherosclerotic vascular disease, was probably non-existent. Not all of this carbohydrate was digestible. As much as 50% of the energy intake for indigenous Australians (Aborigines or Kooris) living on the Victorian Plains was derived from fructo-oligosaccharides of the inulin type, from a tuberous plant known as Murnong (123,124). This was indigestible and fermented in the colon. Prior to

European settlement in Australia, atherosclerotic vascular disease was unknown, yet life expectancies at birth were over 60 years. The question is how much of this cardiovascular protection was attributable to nutrition. Furthermore, how much of this was related to the amount and type of carbohydrate intake ?

Possible effects of dietary carbohydrate on cardiovascular disease

There are a variety of ways in which a high carbohydrate diet might be protective of cardiovascular disease risk:

1. Maintenance of insulin sensitivity - especially in the basal state. High carbohydrate diets tend to lower basal (fasting) glucose and insulin over several days (125). In turn, this decreases risk factors (hyperglycemia and hyperinsulinaemia) for cardiovascular disease.

2. Fermentable carbohydrate in the colon produces absorbable SCFA (short chain fatty acids), with potential regulation of hepatic gluconeogenesis and insulin handling (126). Effects on lipoprotein metabolism are also in evidence (127).

3. Providing companion dietary compounds (micronutrients and phytochemicals) which tend to be protective of the cardiovascular system (128).

4. Displacement of nutritionally disadvantageous components of the diet (e.g. saturated animal fat.

5. Increasing satiety and decreasing the energy density of the diet, making obesity less likely (129-131).

Optimising intake of carbohydrates for CVD protection

Food sources

The food source of carbohydrate may have a bearing on the particular aspect of cardiovascular risk being addressed. Examples of the potential changes in risk with increased intake of particular food carbohydrate sources are shown in Table 11 (arrows show direction of change). Interestingly, whatever the specific effects on cardiovascular risk factors, the sum total of effect on cardiovascular events of increased plant food intake is favourable.

Patterns of eating

If carbohydrate-containing foods are low in fat and consumed as snacks throughout the day, cardiovascular risk is lower (132). More recent reviews of feeding patterns and BMI (body mass index) raise questions about the adequacy of food intake methodology to capture snacking information reliably (133).

Staple foods

One of the major cultural, economic and ecosystem issues relating to food which confronts public health policy-makers is how much carbohydrate should be provided by a staple crop, and how much should come from various other food sources. Populations with a carbohydrate staple such as potatoes, maize, rice or wheat tend to have low CVD rates (134).

Food security, however, would indicate that over-dependence on one crop is not desirable. There is a strong case for food variety to improve cardiovascular risk profiles (135-137).

TABLE 11
Effect of food carbohydrates on cardiovascular risk factors

	Body fatness	Lipoproteins, triglycerides	Blood pressure	Glycemic status	Thrombosis	Antioxidant status	CV events
Cereal	?↓	→	?	↓	?	?	↓
Fruits (not fruit juice)	?↓	→↑		↑→↓	?	↓	
Vegetable	↓	↓	↓	↑→↓		↓	↓
Legumes	?↓	↓		↓	?	?	↓
Nuts	→↑	↓	?		?	↓	↓
Combination*	↓	↓	↓	↓	↓	↓	↓

* The combined effects of these foods is best judged by indices of total plant food intake or variety

Carbohydrates and cancer

Introduction

Interest in the role of carbohydrate in the aetiology of human cancer has been fuelled in recent decades by the debate about the role of dietary fibre in colorectal carcinogenesis. Carbohydrates include sugars and oligosaccharides, starches and non-starch polysaccharides (NSP). In epidemiological studies it is often difficult to distinguish between the effect of the sugars and starches and the role of total energy intake and the associated overweight. An additional problem has been that consumption of a diet rich in, for example, root vegetables, is often associated with low income and poor variety in the diet. Thus there is a range of confounding factors which often make interpretation of epidemiological data difficult.

Carbohydrate, unlike protein or some fats, does not yield potent carcinogens during cooking or storage, and indeed most of the discussion about the role of carbohydrate in human carcinogenesis has concerned cancer prevention in the large bowel. However, there is a clear and indisputable relationship between being overweight and cancers at a number of body sites (138) and, of course, a relationship between consumption of excess energy and being overweight. In those situations where carbohydrate intake has been positively correlated with cancer risk it has been usual to assume that the carbohydrate intake is simply a surrogate measure of excess energy intake resulting in being overweight. There has been much more interest in the possible protective role of carbohydrate, in particular against colorectal cancer. Starting from the premise that colorectal cancer is caused by a luminal carcinogen or promoter formed by bacterial action on some benign substrate (139), it was postulated that dietary fibre protects by:

a. Modifying the colonic bacterial flora to one less likely to produce toxic metabolites;

b. Being itself fermented to yield an environment in the colon less conducive to bacterial production of carcinogens/promoters;

c. Causing stool bulking, thereby decreasing the concentration of luminal carcinogens or promoters; and

d. Speeding the rate of transit of the colonic contents, allowing less time for carcinogens or promoters to act.

Diet has a profound effect on the flora of the caecum (140). Increased dietary fibre results in a non-specific increase in most components of the gut bacterial flora because the enzymes responsible for the breakdown of the macromolecules are largely extracellular (141) and so the released products are available as nutrients to the whole flora. It is not clear, therefore, how this general increase in bacterial population density would decrease the rate of carcinogen production. More recently, non-digestible oligosaccharides like inulin and its hydrolysate oligofructose, have been shown to selectively stimulate the growth of colonic bifidobacteria, opening the way to selectively and significantly modify the composition of the colonic microbiota (142). The major products of bacterial fermentation of carbohydrate are the short chain fatty acids (SCFA), and these acidify the caecum (143). Most of the bacterial enzymes responsible for the production of carcinogens/mutagens have pH optima of 7 or above (138) and so acidification of the caecal lumen would decrease the toxicity of luminal contents to the gut mucosa (144). There is very strong support that dietary fibre protects against colorectal cancer by causing stool bulking, thus decreasing luminal carcinogens or promoters. The greatest effect is seen with wheat bran, and this has been documented by many groups in many countries.

Sugars and oligosaccharides

Sucrose

Since sucrose intake is a significant contributor to total energy intake, it is a standard feature of diet surveys and so there has been a lot of information gathered on its relation to human cancer risk. In general this has shown remarkably little evidence for such a relationship (145). Since sucrose is readily digested, it is a contributor to total energy intake and so might be expected to be associated with those cancers associated with high energy intake, such as colon cancer and the hormone-related cancers, but such an association has not been observed (146).

Lactose

The vast majority of northern Europeans and their descendants worldwide, retain their small bowel lactase throughout their life. Dietary lactose would be well-digested in their small bowel and so would be expected to behave epidemiologically like sucrose. However, the majority of the adult population of the rest of the world is lactose intolerant, having lost their small intestinal lactase during childhood (147). The populations where a high percentage of adults are lactose-tolerant are the only ones in which large bowel cancer is common.

In lactose-intolerant persons, the lactose reaches the large bowel and is fermented to short chain fatty acids (SCFA), thereby contributing to caecal acidification and laxation, and having an effect similar to that of dietary fibre. If dietary fibre is protective against large bowel carcinogenesis then lactose would be expected to also be protective of lactose-intolerant populations (148).

Oligosaccharides

There has been considerable interest in the potential protective effects of fructo-oligosaccharides which are present in some plant foods and are also available commercially. These oligosaccharides are thought to modify the caecal bacterial flora (increasing the numbers of lactobacilli and bifidobacteria, and decreasing the numbers of bacteroides and clostridia) and to acidify the caecum (as a result of rapid fermentation to short chain fatty acids), thereby causing a decreased rate of production of luminal carcinogens/promoters. There is at present, however, only preliminary evidence available which does not permit final evaluation of this interesting hypothesis.

Starches

There have been some studies (149) on the relation between starch intake and colorectal, gastric and breast cancers. Starchy foods in general are associated with an increased risk of these cancers but the correlations may be secondary to other factors. One study of breast cancer indicated that starch was a risk factor in a northern Italian population (150) but considered that starch might only be a marker for total energy intake (which has long been known to be a risk factor for breast cancer). A large study of 23 populations found that starchy foods such as potatoes were inversely correlated with risk of cancers of the colon, breast, prostate and endometrium (146).

Dietary fibre

Burkitt proposed a hypothesis that 'dietary fibre' is a major contributor to protection against colorectal carcinogenesis (139). For the purposes of that hypothesis dietary fibre was defined as the dietary carbohydrate that reaches the large bowel. In the 1970s there were no good assays for dietary fibre and so epidemiologists used intakes of fibre-rich foods as a surrogate measure and obtained results in population studies that showed a very strong protection.

These results were treated as hypothesis-supporting and were followed by a host of case-control studies, which tended to give less convincing support. A major problem with all case-control studies of colorectal cancer is the lack of specificity of the symptoms, which leads to a lag between the onset of symptoms and the actual diagnosis of cancer. Since the presence of symptoms during this lag is likely to cause an insidious change in the diet, it is necessary to use diet recall methods to determine the pre-symptoms diet. Such methods are notoriously inaccurate. This problem was obviated in a prospective study of U.S. nurses, which observed a protective effect of fibre (151).

A further problem with these studies, however, was the method used to determine dietary fibre intake. On the assumption that no starch reaches the colon, methods have been developed to assay non-starch polysaccharides (NSP) and this has been used as a measure of dietary fibre. However, from measures of daily stool weight, we can calculate the amount of carbohydrate that must reach the colon simply to feed the bacteria that make up more than 25% of faeces (152). From this it has been concluded that at least 60-70g carbohydrate reaches the colon per day (153), as compared to the 12-15 g NSP per day used in case-control studies. A proportion of dietary starch is undigested during small bowel transit and so reaches the colon in addition to the NSP (152). Indeed there is probably far more starch than NSP reaching the colon.

In examining whole grain intake in 15 case-control studies, a strong protective effect was observed that was not seen when refined grain was studied (154).   A review of 58 case control or cohort studies found a similar strong protective effect for cereals and cereal fibre, as shown in Table 12.

TABLE 12
Summary of a review of 58 studies of diet and colorectal cancer risk

	Number of papers	Effect on colorectal cancer risk		
		Protection	**No effect**	**Promotion**
Cereal intake	36	23	9	4
Cereal fibre	16	13	3	0

These data strongly suggest that cereals, particularly wheat bran, protect against colorectal carcinogenesis. In support of this conclusion, one study (155) demonstrated that diet intervention to increase intake of wheat bran and decrease fat, although it did not affect the rate of colorectal adenoma formation, it prevented their growth to more than 1cm in diameter. This is the key step in colorectal carcinogenesis (148). Further, a U.S. cohort study (where most of the cereal would have been wheat) showed a strong dose-response effect in the protection by cereal intake (156).

Summary

There is little evidence of any significant correlation between intake of mono-, di- and oligosaccharides and cancer at any site that could not be explained by total energy intake.

There is stronger evidence of a positive correlation between intake of starch or refined carbohydrate and risk of cancers of the colon and breast. This may be because starch intake is a surrogate for total energy intake. There is no good hypothesis to explain why the products of starch digestion (which would be absorbed and delivered to the colon by the vascular route) should be organotropic carcinogens for the colon and breast. Indeed if butyrate has its anticarcinogenic effects (157,158) *in vivo* as well as *in vitro* then a protective effect would have been more likely.

There is still dispute about the protective effect of dietary fibre against colorectal cancer. Since the assay of dietary fibre appears to be very inaccurate it is remarkable that any effect has been seen at all. When better surrogate measures of dietary fibre are used there is much stronger evidence of protection. The data suggest a protective effect for whole grain cereals, particularly wheat (which is much richer in fibre and which has the greatest stool bulking effect).

Carbohydrates and dental caries

Introduction

Dental caries is one of the most widespread oral diseases. Its causation has been associated with food carbohydrates since the beginning of scientific approaches to dental problems. It is still true that eating food containing carbohydrates is a risk factor. Research, especially epidemiology, during the last 25 years, however, has markedly modified current views.

Dental caries - principle of development of lesions

In 1962, three principal factors were defined, all of which are required for the development of carious lesions (177):

1. *Microorganisms* in the mouth with the potential to form acid from carbohydrates.

2. *Substrates* locally available in the mouth as a source of energy for the metabolism of the acidogenic oral bacteria.

3. *Host properties.* The human being is the host for oral microorganisms and the relevant host properties (besides presence of teeth to be colonized by bacteria) are susceptibility to chemo-bacterial attack and protective resistance/defence, as well as the potential for regeneration.

Microorganisms

It is important to realize that microorganisms, such as bacteria, are normal inhabitants of the mouth. Oral bacteria are harmless in thin layers, and are cariogenic only in thick, organized and undisturbed "plaque" on the teeth. This had been shown by measurement of acid formation on the teeth after rinsing with sugar solutions (178). Immediate drops in pH were found when thick plaque was present, whereas after removal of the plaque no acidity could be detected on the cleaned surface. The same phenomenon was reported from a number of laboratories where pH telemetry is used to measure the acidogenic potential of carbohydrate-containing foodstuffs: if the experimenter does not let plaque grow for at least 2 days, no acid formation can be observed (179).

Substrates

In the aetiology of caries, the sources of substrates for cariogenic bacteria are mainly foodstuffs and drinks containing sugars and other carbohydrates. This utilization of some of the food by bacteria is a local side effect in the mouth during food passage, in contrast to the systemic effect of carbohydrates as a source of energy for the host.

It is the result of the side effect, namely acid formation in the bacterial plaque on the teeth, which causes demineralization. The carbohydrates consumed exert no direct damaging effect on the teeth. During sleep and when no food is available, the acidogenic plaque bacteria can metabolize and survive on a minimum supply of substrate derived from carbohydrate sidechains of salivary mucins. At these low substrate concentrations, no cariogenic amounts of acid are formed.

Host factors/properties

Although extremely hard and therefore quite resistant to wear, the enamel covering the tooth crowns is slightly soluble in acids. This fact is the essence of the risks threatening dental health, because eating of food with a certain degree of acidity, as well as drinking of acidic fruit juices and other acidic beverages occurs daily at meals and between meals. Moreover, since a normal diet is rich in carbohydrates, additional acids can be formed if bacterial plaque is present on the teeth.

One way of minimizing these risks from the side of the host is to minimize the frequency of eating and drinking. Other possibilities are to adopt a good oral hygiene habit, to try to increase resistance of teeth against acid, and to improve the repair mechanisms which are provided naturally by secretion of saliva. Saliva contains the buffering bicarbonate system which at least in part can neutralize damaging acids. Moreover, saliva is a solution of calcium and phosphate which at neutrality is oversaturated with respect to enamel apatite. This results in automatic remineralization when, after an acid attack, the pH returns to normal. Such a "normal" remineralization process is very slow, however, and if demineralization is stronger and lasts longer than the time for remineralization, then carious destruction of teeth occurs.

At this point the action of fluoride ions comes in. The presence of fluoride ions protects tooth enamel mineral from becoming demineralized. This protection is only partial, but fluoride ions have a second important capacity - they speed up and improve remineralization and repair. This process requires lifelong frequent tooth-fluoride contacts to maintain dental health. Fluoride sources may be drinking water or tea, or use of a fluoride-containing toothpaste twice a day.

Dietary sugars and caries prevalence

An association between intake of sugars and dental caries was first studied experimentally in the early 1950s on inmates of the Vipeholm asylum in Sweden (180). The Vipeholm Study was the first to reveal the distinction between the effects of amount of sugars eaten, versus the frequency of sugar intake. The experiment showed that restriction of sugar intake to four main meals daily did not significantly increase the caries activity, even if large amounts of sugar (300 g/day) were given. On the other hand, when 8 or 24 between-meal sugar-containing snacks were given daily, caries incidence rose dramatically.

Sugars do not give rise to production of dangerous amounts of acid in the oral cavity when plaque is absent or only present in thin layers. Therefore, it is feasible to separate modern epidemiological research from early findings accumulated in the pre-dental hygiene era. This is the more important because during the same time span in which oral hygiene practice developed, the sale of toothpastes containing fluoride in caries-inhibiting concentrations rose up to more than 95% in many countries.

It is obvious that while dietary sugars are a determinant in the development of caries, they are not the most important factor in the aetiology of the disease. Studies done with groups of children have indicated that frequent consumption of candy did not seem to be a significant determinant of caries, but instead, the oral hygiene status appeared to be the more important caries risk factor (181,182). The Netherlands is one of the developed countries where caries prevalence within the last 25 years has decreased rapidly, although sugar consumption is still more than 90% of what it was in 1965. In Sweden, Norway and New Zealand, sugar consumption between 1982 and 1985 increased, but nevertheless, regular epidemiological monitoring of caries data showed that the caries prevalence in children continued to decrease.

Summary

Although a relationship between sugars and dental caries is accepted by all clinicians and researchers working in the dental field, the degree of emphasis on the importance of this factor in prevention and control of the disease varies. The information we have available today, based on studies into the situation in the 1990s, should allow for a more scientific and rational approach to the role of fermentable carbohydrates in dental caries. If one intended to advise in principle against consumption of all cariogenic food, it would be irrational not to advise, for instance, against consumption of milk and fruit, but only against consumption of sucrose. The recommendation of a varied diet, oral hygiene and fluoride use seems to be the better alternative.

The most important observation emerging from recent epidemiologic studies is that more and more populations are characterized by a decreasing caries prevalence in the young generation, mostly independent from intake of sugars and other carbohydrates. A basic "personal prevention package" of oral hygiene habits - cleaning with a toothbrush and using fluoride toothpaste - is probably sufficient to keep 75 per cent of adolescents caries free. In short, dental health problems do not require any dietary recommendations in addition to, or other than, those required for maintenance of general health.

REFERENCES

1. FAO. 1996. FAOSTAT (PC version) (CD-ROM). Rome.

2. Stoskopf, N.C. 1985. *Cereal grain crops*. Reston Publishing Co., Inc., Reston, VA

3. Dowler, E.A. and Ok Seo, Y.I. 1985. Assessment of energy intake. *Food Policy*, August: 278-88.

4. Gibson, R.S. 1990. *Principles of nutritional assessment*. Oxford University Press, New York.

5. Holland, B., Unwin, I.D. and Buss, D.H. 1988. Cereals and cereal products. Third supplement to McCance and Widdowson's *The composition of foods*. Royal Society of Chemistry, Cambridge.

6. Lorenz, K.J. and Kulp, K. 1991. *Handbook of cereal science and technology*. Marcel Dekker, Inc., New York.

7. FAO. 1995. *Sorghum and millets in human nutrition*. Rome

8. FAO. 1993. *Maize in human nutrition*. Rome.

9. Desmarchelier, J.A. 1991. Economic and political aspects of sugar from an international perspective. In: Gracey, M., Kretchmar, N. and Rossi, E., eds. *Sugars in nutrition*. Raven Press, New York.

10. Fine, B., Heasman, M., and Wright, J. *Consumption in the age of affluence*. London: Routledge, 1996.

11. FAO. 1990. *Roots, tubers, plantains and bananas in human nutrition*. Rome

12. Woolfe, J.A. *The potato in the human diet*. Cambridge, UK: Cambridge University Press, 1987.

13. Palagopalan, C., Padmaja, G., Nanda, S.K., Moorthy, S.N. *Cassava in food, feed and industry*. Boca Raton, F.L: CRC Press, Inc., 1988.

14. Horton, D. Potatoes. *Production, marketing and programs for developing countries*. Boulder, CO: Westview Press, 1987.

15. Holland, B., Unwin, I.D., Buss, D.H. Vegetables, herbs and spices. Fifth supplement to McCance and Widdowson's *The composition of foods*. Cambridge, UK: Royal Society of Chemistry, 1991.

16. Holland, B., Unwin, I.D., Buss,, D.H. Fruit and nuts. First supplement to the fifth edition of McCance and Widdowson's *The composition of foods*. Cambridge, UK: Royal Society of Chemistry, 1992.

17. Santé Québec. Les Québécoises et les Québécois mangent - ils mieux? *Rapport de l'enquête québécoise sur la nutrition*. Montréal: Gouvernement du Québec, 1995.

18. Morgan, K.J., Zabik, M.E. Amount and food sources of total sugar intake by children ages 5 to 12 years. *American Journal of Clinical Nutrition* 1981;34:404-13.

19. Grigg, D. International variations in food consumption in the 1980's. *Geography* 1993; 78:251-66.

20. Grigg, D. The starchy staples in world food consumption. *Annals of the Association of American Geographers* 1996; 86:412-431.

21. Stephen, A.M., Sieber, G.M., Gerster, Y.A., Morgan, D.R. Intake of carbohydrate and its components - international comparisons, trends over time and effects of changing to low fat diets. *American Journal of Clinical Nutrition* 1995;62:851S-67S.

22. Stephen, A.M. Are high carbohydrate intakes healthy? *Carbohydrates and Health - New Insights. Sydney, Australia*: ILSI, 1995.

23. Wursch, P. Starch in human nutrition. *World Review of Nutrition and Dietetics* 1989; 60:199-256.

24. American Heart Association. Position statement. Dietary guidelines for healthy American adults. A statement for physicians and health professionals by the Nutrition Committee, American Heart Association. *Circulation* 1986;74:1465A-8A.

25. Department of Health. Dietary reference values for food energy and nutrients for the United Kingdom. Report of the panel on dietary reference values of the Committee on Medical Aspects of Food Policy. *Report on Health and Social Subjects* 41. London: HMSO, 1991.

26. Health and Welfare Canada. Actions towards healthy eating Canada's guidelines for healthy eating and recommended strategies for implementation. *The report of the communications/implementation committee*. Ottawa: Canadian Government Publishing Centre, 1991.

27. National Health and Medical Research Council. *Dietary guidelines for Australians*. Canberra: Australian Government Publishing Service, 1992.

28. Cassidy A., Bingham, S.A., Cummings, J.H. Starch intake and colorectal cancer risk: an international comparison. *British Journal of Cancer* 1994;69:937-42.

29. Bright-See, E., Jazmaji, V. Estimation of the amount of dietary starch available to different populations. *Canadian Journal of Physiology and Pharmacology* 1991;60:56-9.

30. Dyssler, P., Hoftem, D. *Estimation of resistant starch intake in Europe*. 1995.

31. Pigman, W. and Horton, D. 1972. Chapter 1. Introduction: structure and stereochemistry of the monosaccharides. In: Pigman, W. and Horton, D., eds. *The carbohydrates: chemistry and biochemistry*, 2nd Edition. Vol 1A, pp. 1-67. Academic Press, New York.

32. Southgate, D.A.T.. 1995. The elusive definition of carbohydrates. In: *Carbohydrates and health: new insights, new directions*. pp. 2-8. International Life Sciences Institute (ILSI) Australasia Inc., Werribee, Victoria. ISBN 0 9586453 0 2.

33. Asp, N-G. 1994. Nutritional classification and analysis of food carbohydrates. *American Journal of Clinical Nutrition* 59 (suppl):679S.

34. Lloyd, N.E. and Nelson, W.J. 1984. Chapter XXI. Glucose- and fructose-containing sweeteners from starch. In: Whistler, R.L., BeMiller, J.N. and Paschall, E.F., eds. *Starch: chemistry and technology*, 2nd edition, p. 611.

35. Chinachoti, P. 1995. Carbohydrates: Functionality in foods. *American Journal of Clinical Nutrition* 61 (suppl.):922S.

36. Asp, N-G.. 1995. Classification and methodology of food carbohydrates as related to nutritional effects. *American Journal of Clinical Nutrition* 61 (suppl.):930S.

37. Bornet, F.R.J. 1994. Undigestible sugars in food products. *American Journal of Clinical Nutrition* 59 (suppl.):763S.

38. Smith, P.S. 1982. Starch derivatives and their use in foods. In: *Food carbohydrates*, Lineback, D.R. and Inglett, G.E., eds., p. 237. AVI Publishing Co., Westport, CT.

39. Lineback, D.R. and Rasper, V.F. 1988. Wheat carbohydrates. In: *Wheat: chemistry and technology,* Y. Pomeranz, ed., Vol. 1, p. 277. American Association of Cereal Chemists, St. Paul, MN.

40. Anderson, J.W. and Bridges, S.R. 1993. Hypocholesterolemic effects of oat bran in humans. In: *Oat bran*, P. J. Wood, ed., p. 139. American Association of Cereal Chemists, St. Paul, MN.

41. Muir, J.G., Young, G.P., O'Dea, K., Cameron-Smith, D., Brown, I.L., and Collier, G.R. 1993. Resistant starch - the neglected 'dietary fiber'? Implications for health. *Dietary fiber bibliography and reviews* 1:33.

42. Englyst, H.N., Kingman, S.M. and Cummings, J.H. 1993. Resistant starch: measurement in foods and physiological role in man. In: *Plant polymeric carbohydrates*, Meuser, F., Manners, D.J., and Seibel, W., eds., p. 137. The Royal Society of Chemistry, Cambridge, U.K.

43. Asp, N-G., Schweizer, T.F., Southgate, D.A.T., and Theander, O., 1992. Dietary fiber analysis, in *Dietary fiber - A component of food: nutritional function in health and disease*. Schweizer, T.F. and Edwards, C.A., eds. Springer-Verlag, London, England.

44. Lee, S. C. and Prosky, L., Dietary fiber analysis for nutrition labeling, *Cereal Foods World* 1992, 37:765-771.

45. AOAC International. 1995.. Total, soluble and insoluble dietary fiber in foods. AOAC official method 991.43. *Official Methods of Analysis*, 16th ed.

46. Selvendran, R.R. and Robertson, J.A. 1990. In: *Dietary fibre: chemical and biological aspects*. Royal Society of Chemistry Special Publication No. 83. Southgate, D.A.T., Waldron, K., Johnson, I.T. and Fenwick, G.R., eds. Royal Society of Chemistry 27-43.

47. Englyst, H.N. and Hudson, G.J., 1987. Colorimetric method for routine measurement of dietary fibre as non-starch polysaccharides. A comparison with gas-liquid chromatography. *Food Chemistry*, 24: 63-76.

48. Englyst, H.N., Quigley, M.E. and Hudson, G.J. 1994. Determination of dietary fibre as non-starch polysaccharides with gas-liquid chromatographic, high-performance liquid chromatographic or spectrophotometric measurement of constituent sugars. *Analyst* 119:1497-1509.

49. Englyst, H.N., Kingman, S.M., and Cummings, J.H. 1992. Classification and measurement of nutritionally important starch fractions. *European Journal of Clinical Nutrition* 46(S2):S33-S50.

50. Champ, M., 1992. Determination of resistant starch in foods and food products: interlaboratory study. *European Journal of Clinical Nutrition* 46(S2):S51-S62.

51. Champ, M., Noah, L., Loizeau, G., and Kozlowski, F., 1997., In: *Complex carbohydrates in foods: definition, functionality, and analysis*. Cho, S., Prosky, L. and Dreher, M., eds. Marcel Dekker Co. In Press.

52. Nyman, M., Pålsson, K.E., Asp, N-G. Effects of processing on dietary fibre in vegetables. *Lebensm Wiss u Technol* 1987, 20, 29-36.

53. Svanberg, M., Nyman, E.M.G.L., Andersson, R., Nilsson, T. Effects of boiling and storage on dietary fibre and digestible carbohydrates in various cultivars of carrots. *Journal of the Science of Food and Agriculture* 1997, 73, 245-254.

54. Oliviera, F.A.R., Lamb, J. The mass transfer process of water, soluble solutes and reducing sugars in carrot cortex tissue. In: *Food properties and computer-aided engineering of food processing systems*. Singh R.P, Medina A.G., eds. Kluwer Academic Publishers, Dordrecht, 1989, pp. 497-502.

55. Bornet, F.R.J. Undigestible sugars in food products. *American Journal of Clinical Nutrition* 1994;59 (suppl), 763S-769S.

56. Hagander, B., Björck, I., Asp, N-G, Efendic, S., Holm, J., Nilsson-Ehle, P., Lundquist, I., Scherstén, B. (1987) Rye products in the diabetic diet- postprandial glucose and hormonal responses in non-insulin-dependent diabetics as compared to starch availability in vitro and rat experiments, *Diabetes Research and Clinical Practice* 3:85.

57. Granfeldt, Y., Hagander, B., Björck, I. (1995) Metabolic responses to starch in oat and wheat products. On the importance of food structure, incomplete gelatinization or presence of viscous fibre, *European Journal of Clinical Nutrition* 49: 189-199.

58. Eliasson, A-C., Gudmundsson, M. (1996) Starch: Physicochemical and functional properties, Chapter 10, In: *Carbohydrates in food*, A-C. Eliasson, ed. Marcel Dekker Inc., pp. 431- 503.

59. Granfeldt, Y., Björck, I., Hagander, B. (1991) On the importance of processing conditions, product thicknss and egg addition, for the glycemic and hormonal responses to pasta- a comparison with white bread made from pasta ingredients, *European Journal of Clinical Nutrition* 45: 489.

60. Wolever, T.M.S., Jenkins, D.J.A., Kalmusky, J., Giordano, C., Guidici, S., Jenkins, A.L., Thompson, L.U, Wong, G.S., Josse, R.G. (1986) Glycemic response to pasta: effect of surface area, degree of cooking and protein enrichment, *Diabetes Care* 9: 401.

61. Englyst, H., Kingman, S., Cummings, J. (1992) Classification and measurement of nutritionally important starch fractions, *European Journal of Clinical Nutrition*, 46: 33S-50S.

62. Holm, J., Koellreutter, B., Wursch, P. (1992) Influence of sterilization, drying and oat bran enrichment of pasta on glucose and insulin responses in healthy subjects and on the rate and extent of in vitro starch digestion, *Euopean Journal of Clinical Nutrition* 46: 629.

63. Björck, I., Nyman, M., Asp, N-G. Extrusion-cooking and dietary fiber: Effects on dietary fiber content and on degradation in the rat intestinal tract. *Cereal Chemistry* 1984, 61, 174-179.

64. Ralet, M.C., Thibault, J.F., Della Valle, G.. Influence of extrusion-cooking on the structure and properties of wheat bran. *Journal of Cereal Science* 1990, 11, 249-259.

65. Siljeström, M., Westerlund, E., Björck, I., Holm, J., Asp, N-G., Theander, O. The effects of various thermal processes on dietary fibre and starch content of whole grain wheat and white flour. *Journal of Cereal Science* 1986, 4, 315-323.

66. Ralet, M.C., Saulnier, L., Thibault, J.F. Raw and extruded fibre from peahulls. Part II: Structural study of the water-soluble polysaccharides. *Carbohydrate Polymers* 1993, 20, 25-34.

67. Caprez, A., Arrigoni, E., Amadò, R., Neukom, H.. Influence of different type of thermal treatment on the chemical composition and physical properties of wheat bran. *Journal of Cereal Science* 1986, 4, 233-239.

68. Livesey, G. Metabolizable energy of macronutrients. *American Journal of Clinical Nutrition* 1995 62 (suppl):1135S-42S.

69. Southgate, D.A.T. Digestion and metabolism of sugars. *American Journal of Clinical Nutrition* 1995 62 (suppl):203S-11S.

70. Lentze, M.J. Molecular and cellular aspects of hydrolysis and absorption. *American Journal of Clinical* Nutrition 1995;61 (suppl):946S-51S.

71. Riby, J.E., Fujisawa, T., Kretchmer, M. Fructose absorption. *American Journal of Clinical Nutrition* 1993 58 (suppl):748S-53S.

72. Reiser, S., Michaelis, O.E., Cataland, S., O'Dorisio, T.M. Effect of isocaloric exchange of dietary starch and sucrose in humans on the gastric inhibitory polypeptide response to a sucrose load. *American Journal of Clinical Nutrition* 1980;33:1907-11.

73. Jenkins, D.J.A., Wolever, T.M.S., Taylor, R.H., Barker, H.M., Fielden, H., Baldwin, J.M., Bowling, A.C., Newman, H.C., Jenkins, A.L., Goff, D.V. Glycemic index of foods: a physiological basis for carbohydrate exchange. *American Journal of Clinical Nutrition* 1981;34:362-66.

74. Wolever, T.M.S., Jenkins, D.J.A. The use of the glycemic index in predicting the blood glucose response to mixed meals. *American Journal of Clinical Nutrition* 1986;43:167-72.

75. Ha, M-A, Mann, J.I., Melton, L.D., Lewis-Barned, N.J. Calculation of the glycaemic index. *Diabetes, Nutrition and Metabolism, Clinical and Experimental* 1992;5:137-39.

76. Wolever, T.M.S. Comments on Tai's mathematical model. *Diabetes Care* 1994;17:1223-24.

77. Foster-Powell, K., Brand Miller, J. International tables of glycemic index. *American Journal of Clinical Nutrition* 1995;62:871S-93S.

78. Wolever, T.M.S., Jenkins, D.J.A., Jenkins, A.L., Vuksan, V., Wong, G.S., Josse, R.G. Effect of ripeness on the glycaemic response to banana. *Journal of Clinical Nutrition and Gastroenterology* 1988; 3:85-88.

79. Collier, G.R., Wolever, T.M.S., Wong, G.S., Josse, R.G. Prediction of glycemic response to mixed meals in non-insulin dependent diabetic subjects. *American Journal of Clinical Nutrition* 1986:44;349-52.

80. Wolever, T.M.S. The glycemic index: Flogging a dead horse? *Diabetes Care, in press.*

81. Wolever, T.M.S., Jenkins, D.J.A., Jenkins, A.L., Josse, R.G. The glycemic index: methodology and clinical implications. *American Journal of Clinical Nutrition* 1991;54:846-54.

82. Thomas, D.E., Brotherhood, J.R., Brand, J.C. Carbohydrate feeding before exercise: effect of glycemic index. *International Journal of Sports Medicine* 1991;12:180-86.

83. Burke, L.M., Collier, G.R., Hargreaves, M. Muscle glycogen storage after prolonged exercise: effect of the glycemic index of carbohydrate feedings. *Journal of Applied Physiology* 1993;75:1019-23.

84. Burkitt, D.P., Trowell, H.S. 1975. *Refined carbohydrate foods and disease: some implication of dietary fibre*. London: Academic Press.

85. Gibson, G.R., Beatty, E.R., Wang, X., Cummings, J.H. 1995. Selective stimulation of bifidobacteria in the human colon. *Gastroenterology* , 108: 975-982.

86. Gibson, G.R., Wang, X. 1994. Bifidogenic properties of different types of fructo-oligosaccharides. *Food Microbiology*, 11: 491-498.

87. Read, N.W., Eastwood, M.A. 1992. Gastro-intestinal physiology and function. In: *Dietary fibre. A component of food,* T.F. Schweizer, C.A. Edwards, eds. London: Springer-Verlag, pp. 103-117.

88. Dunaif, G., Schneeman, B.O. 1981. The effect of dietary fiber on human pancreatic enzyme activity in vitro. *American Journal of Clinical Nutrition*, 34: 1034-1035.

89. Cherbut, C. 1995. Role of gastrointestinal motility in the delay of absorption by dietary fibre. *European Journal of Clinical Nutrition*, 49: S74-S80.

90. Cummings, J.H. 1993. The effect of dietary fiber on fecal weight and constipation. In: *CRC Handbook of dietary fiber in human nutrition*, Spiller, G.A., ed. Boca Raton: CRC Press, pp. 263-349.

91. Salvador, V., Cherbut, C. 1992. Modulation of gastrointestinal transit time by dietary fibre (Régulation du transit digestif par les fibres alimentaires). *Cahiers de nutrition et de diététique*, 27: 290-297.

92. Cherbut, C. 1995. Effects of short-chain fatty acids on gastrointestinal motility. In: *Physiological and clinical aspects of short-chain fatty acids*, Cummings, J.H., Rombeau J.L., Sakata, T., eds. Cambridge: Cambridge University Press, pp. 191-207.

93. Blundell, J.E., Rogers, P.J. Hunger, hedonics, and the control of satiation and satiety. In: *Chemical senses, Volume 4: appetite and nutrition*. Friedman, M.I., Tordoff, M.G., Kare, M.R., eds. New York: Marcel Dekker, Inc., 1991: 127-48.

94. Anderson, G.H. Sugars, sweetness, and food intake. *American Journal of Clinical Nutrition* 1995;62:195S-202S.

95. Drewnowski, A., Kurth, C., Holden-Wiltse, J., Saari, J. Food preferences in human obesity: carbohydrates versus fats. *Appetite* 1992;18:207-21.

96. Rolls, B.J. Sensory-specific satiety. *Nutrition Reviews* 1986;44:93-101.

97. Rolls, B.J., Hetherington, M. The role of variety in eating and body weight regulation. In: *Handbook of the psychophysiology of human eating*. Shepherd, R., ed. Sussex, England: John Wiley & Sons, 1989: 57-84.

98. Drewnowski, A. Sweetness and obesity. In: *Sweetness*. Dobbing, J, ed. Berlin: Springer-Verlag, 1987: 177-92.

99. Mela, D.J. Eating behaviour, food preferences and dietary intake in relation to obesity and body-weight status. *Proceedings of the Nutrition Society* 1996;55: 803-16.

100. Granfeldt, Y., Liljeberg, H., Drews, A., Newman R, Bjorck I. Glucose and insulin responses to barley products: influence of food structure and amylose-amylopectin ratio. *American Journal of Clinical Nutrition* 1994;59:1075-82.

101. Raben, A., Tagliabue, A., Christensen, N.J., Madsen, J., Holst, J.J., Astrup, A. Resistant starch. The effect on postprandial glycemia, hormonal response, and satiety. *American Journal of Clinical Nutrition* 1994;60:544-51.

102. Levine, A.S., Billington, C.J. Dietary fiber: does it affect food intake and body weight? In: *Appetite and body weight regulation: Sugar, fat, and macronutrient substitutes.* Fernstrom, J.D., Miller, G.D., eds. Boca Raton, Florida: CRC Press, Inc., 1994: 191-200.

103. Delargy, H.J., Burley, V.J., O'Sullivan, K.R., Fletcher, R.J., Blundell, J.E. Effects of different soluble:insoluble fibre ratios at breakfast on 24-h pattern of dietary intake and satiety. *European Journal of Clinical Nutrition* 1995;49:754-66.

104. Hill, J.O., Pagliassotti, M.J. and Peters, J.C. Nongenetic determinants of obesity and fat topography. In: *Genetic determinants of obesity*, ed. C. Bouchard. Boca Raton: CRC Press, Inc. 35-48, 1994.

105. Schwarz, J.M., Neese, R.A., Turner, S., Dare, D., Hellerstein, M.K. Short-term alterations in carbohydrate energy intake in humans - Striking effects on hepatic glucose production, de novo lipogenesis, lipolysis, and whole-body fuel selection. *Journal of Clinical Investigation* 96:2735-2743, 1995.

106. Hudgins, L.C., Hellerstein, M., Seidman, C., Neese, R., Diakun, J., Hirsch, J. Human fatty acid synthesis is stimulated by a eucaloric low fat, high carbohydrate diet. *Journal of Clinical Investigation* 97:2081-2091, 1996.

107. Horton, T.J., Drougas, H., Brachey, A., Reed, G.W., Peters, J.C., Hill, J.O. Fat and carbohydrate overfeeding in humans: Different effects on energy storage. *American Journal of Clinical Nutrition* 62:19-29, 1995.

108. Hill, J.O., Peters, J.C., Reed, G.W., Schlundt, D.G., Sharp, T., Greene, H.L. Nutrient balance in humans: Effects of diet composition. *American Journal of Clinical Nutrition* 54:10-17, 1991.

109. Flatt, J.P. Assessment of daily and cumulative carbohydrate and fat balances in mice. *Journal of Nutritional Biochemistry* 2:193-202, 1991.

110. Hill, J.O., Prentice, A.M. Sugar and body weight regulation. *American Journal of Clinical Nutrition* 62:264S-274S, 1995.

111. West, K.M. *Epidemiology of diabetes and its vascular lesions*, Elsevier, New York, 1978.

112. Peterson, D.B., Lambert, J., Gerring, S., Darling, P., Carter, R.D., Jelfs, R., Mann, J.I. Sucrose in the diet of diabetic patients - just another carbohydrate? *Diabetologia* 1986; 29: 216-220.

113. Trowell, H.C. Dietary-fibre hypothesis of the etiology of diabetes mellitus. *Diabetes* 1975; 24: 762-765.

114. Feskens, E.J.M., Bowles, C.H., Kromhout, D. Carbohydrate intake and body mass index in relation to the risk of glucose intolerance in an elderly population. *American Journal of Clinical Nutrition* 1991; 54: 136-140.

115. Mann, J.I. Lines to legumes: changing concepts of diabetic diets. *Diabetic Medicine* 1984; l: 191-198.

116. Brand, J.C., Colagiuri, S., Crossman, S., Allen, A., Roberts, D.C., Truswell, A.S. Low-glycemic index foods improve long-term glycemic control in NIDDM. *Diabetes Care* 1991; 14: 95-101.

117. Snowdon, D.A., Phillips, R.L. Does a vegetarian diet reduce the occurrence of diabetes? *American Journal of Public Health* 1985; 75: 507-512.

118. Bennett, P.H., Knowler, W.C., Baird, H.R. *et al.* Diet and the development of non-insulin-dependent diabetes mellitus: An epidemiological perspective. In: Pozza G. *et al* eds. *Diet, diabetes, and atherosclerosis.* New York, Raven Press, 1984, pp. 109-119.

119. American Diabetes Association. Nutrition recommendations and principles for people with diabetes mellitus. *Diabetes Care* 1994; 17: 519-22.

120. Diabetes and Nutrition Study Group (DNSG) of the European Association for the Study of Diabetes (EASD). Recommendations for the nutritional management of patients with diabetes mellitus. *Diabetes, Nutrition and Metabolism* 1995; 8: 1-5.

121. Crapo, P.A., Reaven, G.M., Olefsky, J.M. Plasma glucose and insulin responses to orally administered simple and complex carbohydrates. *Diabetes* 1976; 25: 741-747.

122. Eaton, S.B. and Konner, M. Paleolithic nutrition. A consideration of its nature and current implications. *New England Journal of Medicine* 1985; 312(5):283-289.

123. Gott, B. Ecology of root use by the Aborigines of southern Australia. *Archaeology Oceania* 1982; 17:59-67.

124. Gott, B. Murnong-Microseris scapigera: a study of a staple food of Victorian Aborigines. *Australian Aboriginal Studies* 1983; 2:2-18.

125. Simpson, R.W., McDonald, J., Wahlqvist, M.L., Balasz, N., Sissons, M. and Atley, L. Temporal study of metabolic change when non-insulin dependent diabetics changed from a low to high carbohydrate-fibre diet. *American Journal of Clinical Nutrition,* 48:104-9, 1988.

126. Topping, D.L. and Wong, S.H. Preventive and therapeutic aspects of dietary fibre. In: *Medical practice of preventive nutrition.* pp. 179-198. Edited by Mark L. Wahlqvist, Jitka S. Vobecky. Smith-Gordon & Co Ltd, London, 1994.

127. Mirsuoka, T., Hata, Y., Takahashi, Y. Effects of long term intake of Neosugar on intestinal flora and serum lipids. In: *Proceedings 3rd Neosugar Research Conference,* Tokyo, Meija-Seika Publications.

128. Truswell, A.S. Protective plant foods: new opportunities for health and nutrition. *Food Australia* 1997; 49(1):40-43.

129. Holt, S. The satiating effects of macronutrients - implications for weight control. *Proceedings of the Nutrition Society of Australia* 1996; 20:47-59.

130. Holt, S., Brand Miller, J.C., Petcoz, P. Relationships between satiety and plasma glucose and insulin responses to foods. *Proceedings of the Nutrition Society of Australia* 1996; 20:177.

131. Holt, S.H.A., Brand MIller, J.C., Petocz, P. and Farmakalidis, E. A satiety index of common foods. *European Journal of Clinical Nutrition* 1995; 49:675-690.

132. Jenkins, D.J.A., Wolever, T.M.S., Vuksan, V., Brighenti, F., Cunnane, S.C., Rao, A.V, Jenkins, A.L., Buckley, G., Patten, R., Singer, W., Corey, P. and Josse, R.G. Nibbling versus gorging: metabolic advantages of increased meal frequency. *New England Journal of Medicine* 1989; 321:929-934.

133. Summerbell, C.D., Moody, R.C., Shanks, J., Stock, M.J. and Geissler, C. Relationship between feeding pattern and body mass index in 220 free-living people in four age groups. *European Journal of Clinical Nutrition* 1996; 50:513-519.

134. Temple, N.J. and Burkitt, D.P. *Western diseases. Their dietary prevention and reversibility.* Humana Press, Totowa, New Jersey, 1994.

135. Hodgson, J.M., Hsu-Hage, B.H-H, Wahlqvist, M.L. Food variety as a quantitative descriptor of food intake. *Ecology of Food and Nutrition* 1994; 32:137-148.

136. Hodgson, J.M., Hage, B.H., Wahlqvist, M.L., Kouris-Blazos, A., Lo, C.S. Development of two food variety scores as measures for the prediction of health outcomes. *Proceedings of the Nutrition Society of. Australia,* 16:62, 1991.

137. Kant, A.K., Schatzkin, A., Harris, T.B., Ziegler, R.G. and Block, G. Dietary diversity and subsequent mortality in the First National Health and Nutrition Examination Survey Epidemiologic Follow-up Study. *American Journal of Clinical Nutrition* 1993; 57:434-440.

138. Hill, M.J. (1996). Overweight and cancer. *European Journal of Cancer Prevention* 5: 151-2.

139. Burkitt, D.P. (1971). Epidemiology of cancer of the colon and rectum. *Cancer* 28: 3-13.

140. Hill, M.J., Fernandez, F. (1990). Bacterial metabolism, fiber and colorectal cancer. In: *Dietary fiber.* Kritchevsky, D., Bonfield, C., Anderson, J.W., eds. Plenum, New York, pp. 417-30.

141. McFarlane, G.T., Englyst, H.N. (1986). Starch utilization by the human large intestinal microflora. *Journal of Applied Bacteriology* 60: 195-201.

142. Gibson, G.R., Beatty, E.R., Wang, X., Cummings, J.H. 1995. Selective stimulation of bifidobacteria in the human colon by oligofructose and inulin. *Gastroenterology* 108:975-982.

143. Pye, G., Crompton, J., Evans, D.F. *et al* (1987). The effect of dietary fibre supplementation on colonic pH in healthy volunteers. *Gut 28: A1366-7.*

144. Rafter, J.J., Branting, C. (1991). Bile acids - interaction with the intestinal mucosa. *European Journal of Cancer Prevention* 1 (Suppl 2): 49-54.

145. Hill, M.J. (1995). Diet and cancer: a review of the scientific evidence. *European Journal of Cancer Prevention* 4 (Suppl 2): 3-42.

146. Armstrong, B.K., Doll, Rf (1975). Environmental factors and the incidence and mortality from cancer in different countries with special reference to dietary practice. *International Journal of Cancer* 15: 617-31.

147. Dahlquist, A. (1983). Digestion of lactose. In: *Milk Intolerance and Rejection* (ed Delmont J); Karger, Basel, pp. 11-16.

148. Hill, M.J. (1986). *Microbes and Human Carcinogenesis*. Edward Arnold, London.

149. UK Nutrition Epidemiology Group (1993). *Diet and cancer: A review of the epidemiological literature*. The Nutrition Society, London.

150. Franceschi, S., Favero, A., Decarli, A., Negri, E., La Vecchia, C., Ferraroni, M., Russo, A., Salvini, S., (1996). Intakes of macronutrients and risk of breast cancer. *Lancet* 347: 1351-6

151. Willett, W.C., Stampfer, M.J., Colditz, G.A., Rosner, B.A., Speizer, F.E., Amadori, D., Conti, E. (1990). Relation of meat, fat and fiber intake to the risk of colon cancer in a prospective study among women. *New England Journal of Medicine* 323: 1664-72.

152. Stephen, A.M., Haddad, A.C., Phillips, S.F. (1983). Passage of carbohydrate into the colon; direct measurements in humans. *Gastroenterology* 85: 589-95.

153. Stephen, A.M. (1985). Effects of food on the intestinal microflora. In: *Food and the gut* Hunter, J.O., Alun-Jones, V., eds. Balliere Tyndall, London; pp. 57-77.

154. Jacobs, D.R., Slavin, J., Marquart, L. (1995). Whole grain intake and cancer; a review of the literature. *Nutrition and Cancer* 24: 221-9.

155. MacLennan, R., Macrae, F., Bain, C., Battistutta, D., Chapuis, P., Gratten, H., Lambert, J., Newland, R.C., Ngu, M., Russel, A. (1995). Randomised trial of intake of fat, fiber and beta carotene to prevent colorectal adenomas. *Journal of the National Cancer Institute* 87: 1760-6.

156. Thun, M.J., Calle, E.E., Namboodiri, S., Flanders, W.D., Coates, R.J., Byers, T., Boffetta, P., Garfinkel, L., Heath, C.W. Jr. (1992). Risk factors for fatal colon cancer in a large prospective study. *Journal of the National Cancer Institute* 84: 1491-1500.

157. Johnson, I.T. (1995). Butyrate and markers of neoplastic change in the colon. *European Journal of Cancer Prevention* 4: 365-72.

158. Hague, A., Paraskeva, C. (1995). The short chain fatty acid butyrate induces apoptosis in colorectal tumour cell lines. *European Journal of Cancer Prevention* 4: 359-64.

159. Balfour, J.A., McTavish, D. Acarbose: an update of its pharmacology and therapeutic use in diabetes mellitus. *Drugs* 1993;46:1025-54.

160. Jenkins, D.J.A., Wolever, T.M.S. Slow release carbohydrate and the treatment of diabetes. *The Proceedings of the Nutrition Society* 1981;40:227-35.

161. Jenkins, D.J.A., Taylor, R.H., Goff, D.V., Fielden, H., Misiewicz, J.J., Sarson, D.L., Bloom, S.R., Alberti, K.G.M.M. Scope and specificity of acarbose in slowing carbohydrate absorption in man. *Diabetes* 1981;30:951-54.

162. Cummings, J.H., Macfarlane, G.T. The control and consequences of bacterial fermentation in the human colon. *Journal of Applied Bacteriology* 1991;70:443-59.

163. Nordgaard, I., Mortensen, P.B., Langkilde, A.M. Small intestinal malabsorption and colonic fermentation of resistant starch and resistant peptides to short-chain fatty acids. *Nutrition* 1995;11:129-37.

164. Roediger, W.E.W. The place of short-chain fatty acids in colonocyte metabolism in health and ulerative colitis: the impaired colonocyte barrier. In: Cummings, J.H., Rombeau, J.L., Sakata, T., eds. *Physiological and clinical aspects of short-chain fatty acids*. Cambridge University Press, Cambridge, 1995, pp. 337-51.

165. Sakata, T. Effects of short-chain fatty acids on the proliferation of gut epithelial cells *in vivo*. In: Cummings, J.H., Rombeau, J.L., Sakata, T., eds. *Physiological and clinical aspects of short-chain fatty acids*. Cambridge University Press, Cambridge, 1995, pp. 289-305.

166. Wolever, T.M.S., Jenkins, D.J.A. Effect of fiber and foods on carbohydrate metabolism. In: Spiller, G., ed. *Handbook of dietary fiber in human nutrition*, CRC Press Inc., Boca Raton, FL, pp. 111-162.

167. Jenkins, D.J.A., Wolever, T.M.S., Leeds, A.R., Gassull, M.A., Dilawari, J.B., Goff, D.V., Metz, G.L., Alberti, K.G.M.M. Dietary fibres, fibre analogues and glucose tolerance: importance of viscosity. *British Medical Journal* 1978;1:1392-94.

168. Wood, P., Braaten, J., Scott, F.W., Riedel, K.D., Wolynetz, M.S., Collins, M.W. Effect of dose and modification of viscous properties of oat gum on plasma glucose and insulin following an oral glucose load. *British Journal of Nutrition* 1994;72:731-43.

169. Wolever, T.M.S. In vitro and in vivo models for predicting the effect of dietary fiber and starchy foods on carbohydrate metabolism. In: Kritchevsky, D., Bonfield, C., eds. *Dietary fiber in health and disease*. Eagan Press, St. Paul, MN, 1995, pp. 360-77.

170. Gordon, D.T. Total dietary fiber and mineral absorption. In: Kritchevsky, D., Bonfield, C., Anderson, J.W., eds. *Dietary fiber: chemistry, physiology and health effects*. Plenum Press, New York, 1990, pp. 105-28.

171. Kelsay, J.L. Effects of fiber on vitamin bioavailability. In: Kritchevsky, D., Bonfield, C., Anderson, J.W., eds. *Dietary fiber: chemistry, physiology and health effects*. Plenum Press, New York, 1990, pp. 129-35.

172. Trinidad, T.P., Wolever, T.M.S., Thompson, L.U. Availability of calcium for absorption in the small intestine and colon from diets containing available and unavailable carbohydrates: an in vitro assessment. *International Journal of Food Sciences and Nutrition* 1996;47:83-88.

173. Trinidad, T.P., Wolever, T.M.S., Thompson, L.U. The effect of acetate and propionate on calcium absorption from the rectum and distal colon of humans. *American Journal of Clinical Nutrition* 1996;63:574-78.

174. Glinsmann, W.H., Park, Y.K. (1995). Perspective on the 1986 Food and Drug Administration assessment of the safety of carbohydrate sweeteners: uniform definitions and recommendations for future assessments. *American Journal of Clinical Nutrition* 62 (1 Suppl), 161S-168S.

175. Clutton, A. (1994). Sweetness with no extra waist. *Food Processing* July, 27-30.

176. Ackermann, L.G.J. (1990). *Structure elucidation of and synthetic approaches to monatin, a metabolite from sclerochiton ilicifolius.* Ph.D. Thesis, University of Stellenbosch, Stellenbosch, 1--164.

177. Keyes, P.H. Recent advances in dental caries research: Bacteriology. *International Dental Journal* 1962;12:443-464.

178. Stephan, R.M., Miller, B.F. A quantitative method for evaluating physical and chemical agents which modify production of acids in bacterial plaques on human teeth. *Journal of Dental Research* 1943;22:45-51.

179. Imfeld, T. *Identification of low-risk dietary components.* Basel, Karger, 1983.

180. Gustafson, B., Quensel, C., Lanke, L., *et al.* The Vipeholm dental caries study: the effect of different carbohydrate intake on caries activity in 436 individuals observed for five years. *Acta Odontologica Scandanavica* 1954;11:232-64.

181. Palin-Palokas, T., Hausen, H., Heinonen, O. Relative importance of caries risk factors in Finnish mentally retarded children. *Community Dentistry and Oral Epidemiology* 1987;15:19-23.

182. Pulgar-Vidal, O., Schr der, U. Dental health status in Latin-American preschool children in Malm . *Swedish Dental Journal* 1989; 13:103-109.

183. Devlin, J.T., Williams, C. Foods, Nutrition and Sports Performance; a final consensus statement. *Journal of Sports Sciences* 1991; 9 (Suppl 9):iii.

184. Ahlborg, B., Bergstrom, J., Brohult, J., Ekelund, L-G., Hultman, E., Maschio, G. Human muscle glycogen content and capacity for prolonged exercise after different diets. *Forsvarsmedicin* 1967;3:85-99.

185. Hermansen, L., Hultman, E., Saltin, B. Muscle glycogen during prolonged severe exercise. *Acta Physiologica Scandinavica* 1967;71:129-139.

186. Costill, D.L., Gollnick, P.D., Jansson, E.D., Saltin, B., Stein, E.M. Glycogen depletion pattern in human muscle fibres during distance running. *Acta Physiologica Scandinavica* 1973;89:374-383.

187. Gollnick, P.D., Armstrong, R.B., Saubert, I.V.C.W., Sembrowich, W.L., Shepherd, R.E., Saltin, B. Glycogen Depletion patterns in human skeletal muscle fibers during prolonged work. *Pfluegers Archives* 1973;344:1-12.

188. Bergstrom, J., Hermansen, L., Hultman, E., Saltin, B. Diet, muscle glycogen and physical performance. *Acta Physiologica Scandinavica* 1967;71:140-150.

189. Sherman, W., Costill, D., Fink, W., Miller, J. Effect of exercise-diet manipulation on muscle glycogen and its subsequent utilization during performance. *International Journal of Sports Medicine* 1981;114:114-118.

190. Brewer, J., Williams, C., Patton, A. The influence of high carbohydrate diets on endurance running performance. *European Journal of Applied Physiology* 1988;57:698-706.

191. Williams, C., Brewer, J., Walker, M. The effect of a high carbohydrate diet on running performance during a 30-km treadmill time trial. *European Journal of Applied Physiology* 1992;65:18-24.

192. Gaitanos, G.C., Williams, C., Boobis, L.H., Brooks, S. Human muscle metabolism during intermittent maximal exercise. *Journal of Applied Physiology* 1993;75:712-719.

193. Essen, B., Kaijser, L. Regulation of glycolysis in intermittent exercise in man. *Journal of Physiology* 1978;281:499-511.

194. Jacobs, I., Westlin, N., Karlsson, J., Rasmusson, M., Houghton, B. Muscle glycogen and diet in elite soccer players. *European Journal of Applied Physiology* 1982;48:297-302.

195. Horowitz, J.F., Coyle, E.F. Metabolic responses to pre-exercise meals containing various carbohydrates and fat. *American Journal of Clinical Nutrition* 1993;58:235-41.

196. Thomas, D., Brotherhood, J., Brand, J. Carbohydrate feeding before exercise: Effects of glycemic index. *International Journal of Sports Medicine* 1991;12:180-186.

197. Okano, G., Sato, Y., Takumi, Y., Sugawara, M. Effect of ∠h pre-exercise high carbohydrate and high fat meal ingestion on endurance performance and metabolism. *International Journal of Sports Medicine.* 1996;17:530-534.

198 Pascoe, D.D., Costill, D.L., Robergs, R.A., Davis, J.A., Fink, W.J., Pearson, D.R. Effects of exercise mode on muscle glycogen restorage during repeated days of exercise. *Medicine and Science in Sports and Exercise* 1990; 22:593-598.

199. Kirwan, J.P., Costill, D.L., Mitchell, J.B., Houmard, J.A., Flynn, M.G., Fink, W.J., Beltz, J.D. Carbohydrate balance in competitive runners during successive days of intense training. *Journal of Applied Physiology* 1988; 65:2601-2606.

200. Shannon, W.R. (1922) Neuropathologic manifestations in infants and children as a result of anaphylactic reaction to foods contained in their dietary. *American Journal of Diseases of Children* 24:89.

201. Randolph, T.G. (1947) Allergy as a causative factor of fatigue, irritability and behavior problems in children. *Journal of Pediatrics* 31:560.

202. Deutsch, R.M. (1977) *The new nuts among the berries.* Bull Publishing Co. p. 34, 235-238.

203. Speer, F. (1954) The allergic tension-fatigue syndrome. *Pediatric Clinics of North America* 1:1029.

204. Cott, A. (1977) Treatment of learning disabilities. In: William, R.J., Kalita, D.K., eds. *A physician's handbook on orthomolecular medicine.* New York, Pergamon Press 90-91.

205. Wolraich, M.L., Wilson, D.B., White, J.W. (1996) The effect of sugar on behavior or cognition in children: A meta-analysis. *Journal of the American Medical Association.*

206. Sternberg, D.B., Martinez, J., McGaugh, J.L., Gold, P.E. (1985) Age-related memory deficits in rats and mice: enhancement with peripheral injections of epinephrine. *Behavioral and Neural Biology* 44(2):213-20.

207. Gold, P.E. (1986) Glucose modulation of memory storage processing. *Behavioral and Neural Biology* 45(3):342-9.

208. Gonder-Frederick, L.A., Hall, J.L., Vogt, J. (1987) Memory enhancement in elderly humans: effects of glucose ingestion. *Physiology and Behaviour* 41(5):503-4.

209. Manning, C.A., Parsons, M.W., Gold, P.E. (1992) Anterograde and retrograde enhancement of 24 hour memory by glucose in elderly humans. *Behavioral and Neural Biology* 58(2):125-30.

210. Hall, J.L., Gonder-Frederick, L.A., Chewning, W.W., Silveira, J., Gold, P.E. (1989) Glucose enhancement of performance on memory tests in young and aged humans. *Neuropsychologia* 27(9):1129-38.

FAO TECHNICAL PAPERS

FAO FOOD AND NUTRITION PAPERS

Availability: March 1998

Ar – Arabic
C – Chinese
E – English
F – French
P – Portuguese
S – Spanish

Multil – Multilingual
* Out of print
** In preparation

The FAO Technical Papers are available through the authorized FAO Sales Agents or directly from Sales and Marketing Group, FAO, Viale delle Terme di Caracalla, 00100 Rome, Italy.